Contents

A Practical Guide to Leadership Development

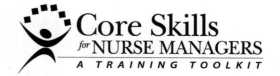

A Practical Guide to

Leadership Development

Skills for Nurse Managers

Patrick R. Coonan, EdD, RN, CNAA

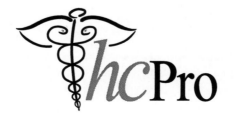

Patrick R. Coonan, EdD, RN, CNAA, Author

Alan H. Cooper, PhD, MBA, Contributing Author

Rebecca Hendren, Senior Managing Editor

Jamie Gisonde, Executive Editor

Emily Sheahan, Group Publisher

Patrick Campagnone, Cover Designer

Mike Mirabello, Senior Graphic Artist

Genevieve d'Entremont, Copyeditor

Sada Preisch, Proofreader

Darren Kelly, Books Production Supervisor

Susan Darbyshire, Art Director

Claire Cloutier, Production Manager

Jean St. Pierre, Director of Operations

Advice given is general. Readers should consult professional counsel for specific legal, ethical, or clinical questions.

Arrangements can be made for quantity discounts. For more information, contact:

HCPro, Inc.
P.O. Box 1168
Marblehead, MA 01945
Telephone: 800/650-6787 or 781/639-1872
Fax: 781/639-2982
E-mail: *customerservice@hcpro.com*

Visit HCPro at its World Wide Web sites: *www.hcpro.com* and *www.hcmarketplace.com*

08/2007
21269

A Practical Guide to Leadership Development

ABOUT THE AUTHORS

Patrick R. Coonan, EdD, RN, CNAA

Dr. Patrick Coonan is the dean and professor of the School of Nursing at Adelphi University in Garden City, NY, and has had a long history of service in nursing service leadership and education. Throughout his career he has held senior patient care management positions at major medical centers in the New York metropolitan area. He has been the chief nursing officer in an academic medical center, a health system, and a teaching community hospital, and completed a fellowship in the Johnson & Johnson–Wharton Fellows Program in Management for Nurse Executives at The Wharton School, University of Pennsylvania. He is certified in Nursing Administration, Advanced, from the American Nurses Association. Dr. Coonan's work now includes leadership assessment and education, integrating technology into nursing management and educational systems, executive coaching, personnel planning with management systems, and organizational analysis and systems implementation.

His academic experience includes administrative and teaching positions at Rutgers University, Long Island University, and Pace University, where he has developed technology-enhanced education programs, and directed and taught informatics and critical care nursing and nursing leadership/management programs. He has held academic administrative positions at the program director level as well as assistant and associate dean positions at Columbia University's School of Nursing.

Dr. Coonan received his EdD and MEd from Columbia University, a master's in Public Administration/Healthcare Administration (MPA) from Long Island University, and a B.S. in Nursing from Adelphi University. He has written and presented extensively on nursing management, leadership, nursing education, and emergency service and response, as well as healthcare management. His research interests include developing academic/service partnerships, improving patient outcomes, and measuring the impact of leadership, management systems, and nursing care on traditional measures such as complications, costs, and personnel issues.

Dr. Coonan is president and principal consultant of Infinite Horizons Consulting, LLC, a consulting firm focused on healthcare and education organizations, specializing in initiatives in planning and implementing educational systems, personnel systems solutions, training and development, and strategic solutions in clinical systems and operations. He can be reached at *pcoonan@ihcllc.com.*

About the contributing author: Alan H. Cooper, PhD, MBA

Alan H. Cooper, PhD, MBA is the vice president for the Center for Learning and Innovation of the North Shore–Long Island Jewish Health System. In this role, Dr. Cooper codeveloped and oversees the leadership development program for a 15-hospital, 35,000-employee integrated health system. He holds an MBA with a concentration in management, and a PhD in experimental psychology with a concentration in human perception and performance. He is an adjunct associate professor at Hofstra University's Frank K. Zarb School of Business and holds a faculty position at the Derner Institute of Advanced Psychological Studies at Adelphi University.

Dr. Cooper is a member of the American Society for Training and Development, the American College of Healthcare Executives, the International Society of Six Sigma Professionals, the American Management Association, the Society for Medical Simulation, and is a senior member of the American Society for Quality.

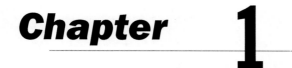

Chapter 1

LEADERSHIP DIMENSIONS AND PROCESSES

Learning objectives

After reading this section, the participant should be able to:

- Differentiate between the roles of manager and leader
- Identify three tasks of leadership

Leadership defined

For many decades, writers have attempted to describe leadership and researchers, through many studies, have attempted to identify the defining characteristics of a leader. The outcome of all this study has led us to one very clear conclusion: Leadership is one of the most observed and least understood phenomena on earth (Burns 1978).

Leadership has been described as multidimensional and multifaceted, as well as a universal human phenomenon that many know when they see it but few can clearly define. There may be almost as many different definitions of leadership as there are people who have attempted to define this. According to Bennis and Nanus (1985):

"Decades of academic analysis have given us more than 350 definitions of leadership. Literally thousands of empirical investigations of leaders have been conducted in the last 75 years alone, but no clear and unequivocal understanding exists as to what distinguishes leaders from nonleaders, and perhaps more important, what distinguishes effective leaders from ineffective leaders."

There is, however, more and more differentiating clarity between the concepts of management and leadership. In most books in the nursing field, there is a considerable amount of focus given to management and very little given to leadership. But we must remember that, unlike management skills, leadership is not necessarily tied to a position. Everyone has the potential to be a leader, and nurses have the responsibility to be leaders in their organizations.

Differences between leadership and management

John Gardner, one of the noted experts in the field of leadership and a prolific author, has outlined nine tasks of leadership that help distinguish it from management. These tasks are:

1. **Envisioning goals:** Pointing others in the right direction in helping the group deal with the tension between long- and short-term goals

2. **Affirming values:** Regenerating and revitalizing the beliefs, values, purposes, and vision shared by members of the group, and challenging the values held by some

3. **Motivating:** Unlocking or channeling motives that exist within members of the group, having and promoting positive attitudes, being creative, and encouraging others to be excited about the future and how they can be a part of it

4. **Managing:** Planning, setting priorities, making decisions, facilitating change, and keeping the system functioning, all in an effort to move the group toward its agreed goals and vision

5. **Achieving a workable unity:** Establishing trust and striving toward cohesion and mutual tolerance while managing conflict

6. **Explaining:** Helping others understand what the vision is, why they are being asked to do certain things, and how they relate to the larger picture

7. **Serving as a symbol:** Serving as a risk taker and acting as the group's source of unity, voice of anger, collective identity, and continuity, as well as its source of hope

8. **Representing the group:** Speaking and acting for or on behalf of the group and being an advocate for the group

9. **Renewing:** Blending continuity and change, and breaking routines, habits, fixed attitudes, perceptions, assumptions, and unwritten rules (Gardner 1989)

Leadership is an art

Leadership is more of an art than a science. Whereas management is often thought of as a science in which a series of logical steps can be followed to implement whatever the role demands, leaders differ from managers in a variety of ways. Leaders are active in formulating goals and objectives for the people who work for them. They look for a better way to do things.

In management, many goals are established by other people and carried out by the managers within the organization. Leaders will act to develop new and fresh approaches to problems that may exist within the organization. Leaders are never satisfied with the status quo. The leader's instinct is to take risks and to challenge those people and ideas within an organization that may be holding it back. Managers work to accomplish the tasks and usually will continue to do whatever is necessary to get the job done without taking on too much risk or moving forward.

Leaders are concerned with relationship building. They promote the people who work for them, help them develop, and move forward. Managers assign people; focus on personnel issues; and focus on how the events get done, how they occur, and how are they accomplished.

It is important to emphasize that a person can be a leader without being in a position of authority. And, as healthcare professionals, every one of us must remember that, because we all have the potential to provide leadership at some point in our life.

Being a leader, not a manager, involves new thinking skills

The purpose of new thinking skills is simple. As a manager you think in logical steps, whereas as a leader the concepts of thinking in new ways may not be logical. In fact, thinking may seem very illogical early on in your leadership development. You will need to take risks, and create new ideas that may be very different.

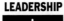

LEADERSHIP

TIP

Get out of the box! Better still, there is no box! Try it.

The purpose of thinking is to collect information and make the best possible use of it. Unfortunately, because of the way our minds work to create fixed concept patterns, we cannot make the best use of new information until we have some means for first restructuring what we have been patterned to learn.

Traditional methods of thinking—such as vertical (also called logical) thinking—taught us to refine such patterns and then establish whether or not they are valid. Most of us are vertical thinkers; in other words, we move forward by sequential steps where each one must be justified. This tends to trap us into thinking in the same way, and consequently we continue to do things the same old way. Learning to think can help us create new patterns and new ways of doing things.

Try lateral thinking: Think from there to here, not here to there

A new way of thinking is lateral thinking, which is concerned with restructuring patterns and looking for new ones. Since we already know how to think vertically, it is important that we learn how to think laterally, because these are complementary. In order to be a good leader, you need to have skills in both of these areas.

(**Note:** An additional method of thinking is called systems thinking, which will be addressed in Chapter 4.)

Lateral thinking is not a new concept; in fact, it is about 40 years old. It essentially has to do with insight, vision, creativity, and humor. Today's healthcare environment requires us to be creative thinkers, as the tremendous changes we face on a daily basis continue to challenge even the best managers and leaders in our systems.

Most of our thinking skills revolve around the fact that we take a conflict, try to look at our history bank to see what has worked before, and then try to find an idea that will move it forward. This system works well when information can be evaluated in some objective manner, but the method does not work well when the new information can be evaluated only through an old idea. Instead of being changed, old ideas are coming out. In fact, old ideas are strengthened and made even more rigid by our validation of trying to figure out how to deal with them. What has worked before will work again.

Lateral thinking is very closely related to creativity. As our healthcare systems become more overloaded and busier, we find that an essential ingredient of change and progress is creativity. We can no longer do things the way that we have always done them, and instead must think creatively. New ideas are the stuff of change and progress in every field, including healthcare. We must begin to think about breaking out of the concept of old ideas, and look at things with a different attitude and approach. Our liberation from old ideas and the stimulation of new ones are some of the aspects of lateral thinking.

LEADERSHIP

TIP

Creativity is an essential part of change. By changing the way you think, you can change the way you look at problems and help develop new solutions.

Another important component of lateral thinking is that you should deliberately seek out irrelevant information, whereas in vertical thinking one selects only what is relevant. As leaders, if we can begin to think laterally as well as vertically, we will be much more creative and have the ability to problem-solve on a different level. It takes work and practice to be able to step out and make the changes necessary for success and to develop the process of lateral thinking. You need to practice in a work setting, and understand the necessary techniques in order to work out all of the details. The ability to think laterally is a much more important skill for a leader than thinking vertically. Again, to contrast the two roles, managers are primarily vertical thinkers, whereas leaders tend to be primarily lateral thinkers. The discussion in Chapter 4 regarding systems thinking will give you a better idea about lateral thinking and its application.

Three major tasks of leadership

Leaders have different tasks depending on their role responsibilities, but some aspects of leadership are common to all roles across healthcare, because they focus on people. Communication, relationship management, and professional development are three of the most important dimensions of leadership, because our industry is so labor intensive. Most of what we do involves people. Whether they are patients or staff, they are still people, and these three aspects are important tools for getting the job done.

Communication and relationship management

When we talk about communication and relationship management, we are discussing the following competencies:

- Labor relation strategies

- Organizational structure and relationships

- Principles of communication and specific applications—for example, crisis communication, alternative dispute resolution, performance improvement, feedback

- Public relations

All of the preceding competencies require one important skill: communication. Effective communication strategies are discussed in detail in Chapter 5, but let's look at some brief issues surrounding these tasks and why they are so important to effective leadership.

Communication and relationship management is the ability to communicate clearly and concisely with both internal and external customers, establish and maintain relationships, and facilitate constructive interactions with individuals and groups.

A Practical Guide to Leadership Development

Building collaborative relationships with the people we work with—and work for—is one of the most important skills that we can develop in communication and relationship management. Collaborative relationships are the cornerstone of healthcare delivery. In today's environment of safety and efficiency, collaborative relationships will only create better patient care outcomes.

LEADERSHIP

TIP

Being a leader is about building relationships. Step out of your comfort zone, take the initiative, and establish some new relationships in your workplace.

One of the ways we can build better collaborative relationships is through effective decision-making. Decision-making is not often discussed in staff meetings. However, staff must make decisions at numerous points. It is the leader's responsibility to ensure that he or she makes appropriate decisions and then move on.

If our staff believes we are unable to make a decision and stick to it, then they will view us as ineffective. Effective leaders make decisions, recognize risks, and identify them to the people who work for them. Sometimes we must act on incomplete information because of the severity of the situation, but always remember that staff will know when complete information is absolutely essential and when you acted on incomplete information inappropriately. This will require us to use our lateral thinking, as described earlier, to come up with creative approaches to solving problems. Arriving at the right solution as a result of competent and creative decision-making is only the first part of the job to build collaborative relationships; the next challenge lies in gaining acceptance of an action or recommended solution. The right solution, kept to yourself, is no good. Leaders have to think through and use a strategy that will result in acceptance of the recommended solution. Strategies include timing, and identifying a proper organizational level or a proper individual to whom the information and solution must be presented.

LEADERSHIP

TIP

Pick a solution and stick to it. It can always be changed later.

Securing involvement and support of appropriate people is important to building the relation-ships that will help carry out decisions. As a leader or a manager in an organization, you can be an effective manager by helping reach a consensus point of view and incorporating solutions that the staff members recommend.

Nurses know how to listen, as we were taught that in school. We also know how to encour-age others to respond effectively and efficiently, and we have been taught how to break down the barriers of communication. Nurse leaders are particularly good at this and should take ad-vantage of the effective communication skills that they already have. Leadership opportunities are frequent in our profession, and not just in management positions. Serving on committees, belonging to a professional association, writing articles for newspapers or professional journals, and so on, are all opportunities for leadership. As discussed earlier when talking about lateral thinking, we are limited only by our imagination and our own willingness to take risks.

Developing staff

Relationship management is connected to the continuous development of the people who work for you and the ongoing renewal of their understanding of what involvement is ex-pected. It is the responsibility of a leader to develop new leaders. We must have visions for the future, and we need to ensure that there are people who will carry out the vision long after we are gone.

Building toward a vision requires collaboration between the leaders and followers. Develop-ment of a significant number of followers who can provide leadership in the absence of a formal leader is just as important as developing new leaders. Succession planning and leader-ship development are discussed in depth in Chapter 10, but briefly, developing others occurs through personal attention, role modeling, precepting, and mentoring.

LEADERSHIP

 Your people are your most important asset. Develop them and they
will develop you.

Personal attention involves the personal guidance given by the leader to another person. It requires that leaders understand the strengths and limitations of the people to whom they

 A Practical Guide to Leadership Development

provide guidance, as leaders need to know what opportunities must be made available, and the expectations to set regarding their contributions to the group.

Role modeling occurs when a more experienced individual performs a role in a way that novices want to follow, whether that concerns style, values, or behavior. You can be a role model without even knowing it. This method of development is essentially a more passive approach.

Precepting is a strategy often used in nursing in which an experienced individual teaches, guides, and assists another in learning a role. Preceptor relationships usually have a specific time limitation, and goals and objectives are clearly outlined between both the preceptor and the preceptee.

Mentoring, in comparison to precepting, is a purposeful relationship in which an experienced, accomplished individual chooses to enter into a relationship with someone with less experience. To have a successful mentoring relationship there must be a match between what the mentor and the mentee want to accomplish. Mentors will open doors for their protégés and give them feedback and guidance about goals and other significant matters in their lives.

 LEADERSHIP

 TIP

Be the person you want them to be. Be the model; make it work!

One of the most important leadership communication skills is to ensure that everybody is on the same page. Keeping an organization's staff on target and focused on the mission is a difficult yet critical task. It is the leader's job to continually test, challenge, and extend personal and collective relationships with staff throughout the process of trying to change behavior. When things get difficult or grind to a halt, the leader's only resource may be the personal relationships that he or she has developed during this process. Identifying with the staff and their concurrent difficulties is critical to maintaining relationships.

References

Burns, J. M. (1978). *Leadership.* New York: Harper Torchbooks.

Bennis, W., and Nanus, B. (1985). *Leaders: The Strategies for Taking Charge.* New York: Harper and Row.

Gardner, J. W. (1989). "The Tasks of Leadership." In W. E. Rosenbach and R. L. Taylor (Eds.), *Contemporary Issues in Leadership* (2nd ed.) Boulder, CO: Westview Press, pp. 24–33.

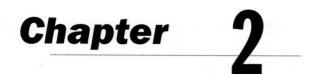

Chapter 2

LEADERSHIP ISSUES IN THE HEALTHCARE ENVIRONMENT

Learning objectives

After reading this section, the participant should be able to:

- Identify key leadership issues in the healthcare environment
- Identify the necessary competencies for being a healthcare leader

What's going on around you

Successful leaders must demonstrate an understanding of the healthcare system and the environment in which healthcare managers and providers function. In this domain, leadership encompasses a long list of core knowledge competencies.

This chapter contains an overview of some of the competencies regarding knowledge of the healthcare environment that leaders need to know and includes some practical approaches for acquiring them. These competencies were developed by the Healthcare Leadership Alliance in 2006 as a way to help healthcare leaders meet the challenges of today's healthcare systems. The competencies were based on job analysis and input from top professional societies, including the American Organization of Nurse Executives (HLA 2006). Discussion of competencies related to professionalism, business knowledge and skills developed by the Healthcare Leadership Alliance will be covered in Chapter 3. Other competencies are discussed throughout the book. You can view the full competency directory at *www.healthcareleadershipalliance.org.*

Community standards of care

In providing leadership in any particular institution—whether it is inpatient, outpatient, or other private facility—nurse leaders must know what the standards of care for that particular community are in order to be competitive and deliver the standards that the community expects.

LEADERSHIP

TIP

All healthcare is local. Know what your community needs and wants.

Regulatory and administrative environment

Leaders need to understand the regulatory and administrative environment in which the organization functions. In this particular area, leaders must be aware of federal rules and regulations, current labor law, and contracts within your organization. Additionally, you must know about accreditation issues and any other external factors that impact your functioning in a leadership role within the organization.

Role of nonclinical professionals

What roles do nonclinical professionals play in the healthcare system? Do you understand how they integrate into your position and the area you manage? Global understanding of the role of all staff within an organization will assist you in using them effectively to deliver patient care when necessary.

Interrelationship between access, quality, cost, resource allocation, accountability, and community

How do these external factors affect the delivery of patient care in your area? All of these parameters are interrelated to the total delivery of patient care. Patients must have access, you must deliver a quality product at the right cost, and you cannot overallocate or under-allocate

 A Practical Guide to Leadership Development

resources to that delivery. You are accountable for it and for what the community thinks about your delivery of services.

The patient perspective

Do you carry out customer service surveys in your organization? What is the patient's perspective of the care that you deliver within your organization? Is your unit performing higher or lower than other units? How often do you actually talk to the patient? All of these perspectives are important for delivering a quality product. The patients are our customers, and if we do not deliver a quality product, or at least one that is perceived as quality by the patients, then we will no longer be competitive.

Workforce issues

This broad subject takes in union issues, staff satisfaction, turnover, retention, and other factors that affect patient care. Maintaining a workforce that is satisfied and that provides quality care is a significant competency that you need to deliver as a leader in any healthcare organization. Workforce issues are varied and can come in many shapes and forms, such as a labor action or just having a small problem with one employee. Workforce issue resolution comes with practice, and involves dealing with history and past practice issues that come from organized labor. Many organizations do not have organized labor, but nonetheless must treat employees fairly and equitably in order to avoid workforce issues.

LEADERSHIP

TIP

Befriend your local nursing school and faculty. The more cooperative you are, the more students they will send.

Corporate compliance

Corporate compliance laws and regulations (for example, physician recruitment, billing and coding practices, antitrust laws, conflicts of interest) can get healthcare leaders into trouble very easily and quickly. Understanding the corporate compliance regulations in your state and practice environment is important to your success as a leader. Today's corporate environment, along with the downfall of some chief executive officers, has increased the federal government's scrutiny of corporate compliance laws. You need to understand how the corporate compliance regulations apply to you as well as your staff.

Education funding

Today's nursing shortage has created a government awareness that has increased funding for nursing education and development. It is the responsibility of nurse leaders to understand what funding is available to improve their own skills or the skills of their staff. Collaboration with human resources and local academic institutions can usually provide insight as to what type of funding might be available. The pursuit of further education is a leadership mandate. Improvement of one's skills and those of the staff are part of leadership's responsibility in moving forward.

Funding

As a leader in healthcare, you must understand where the money comes from and the funding and payment mechanisms of the healthcare system. In particular, you need to understand how you can help generate reimbursement, and how your staff can contribute to either positive or negative cash flow of your organization. Funding and payment become more and more complicated every year. Continuous education of a leader in understanding the payment mechanism of healthcare is fundamental to the success of the position. Any clinical leader who can discuss finance with the finance people and administrators of the organization will be highly regarded as someone who understands the system and is a contributor to the success of that system. The expression "you must walk the walk and talk the talk" is extremely important in understanding financial ramifications and reimbursement mechanisms within healthcare. Continuous education and knowledge gained on the outside through newsletters, newspapers, government publications, and Web sites will keep you informed about the financial payment mechanisms of the system.

Global healthcare trends

A working knowledge of issues affecting global health is mandatory for a leader in any healthcare organization. Global healthcare issues, trends, and perspectives—such as aging populations, insurance costs, malpractice issues, nursing shortages, nursing faculty shortages, and so on—affect you directly as a leader in the healthcare organization. The aging population and the increasing demand for services as the baby boomer population ages, topped off by a nursing shortage, will affect how you operate and how the staff in your unit operates. How will you be able to deliver effective care to an increasing, and increasingly ill, population when you have fewer nurses? As the nursing shortage proliferates, nurses will demand higher salaries. This coupled with an aging and sicker population means that there will be more hospitalization for the aging population of our world over the next 10 to 20 years.

Conversely, with decreasing reimbursements for nursing services and to hospitals in general, how will you as a nursing leader be able to deliver quality, effective services to an increasing population of elderly people over time? This will require true leadership and creative thinking and a review of how we actually deliver services.

Governmental, regulatory, and accreditation agencies

To maintain a quality environment, nurse leaders must know what governmental, regulatory, professional, and accreditation agencies will regulate their practice environment and their requirements for successful accreditation. The Joint Commission, the Centers for Medicare & Medicaid Services (CMS), and other local and national regulatory and accreditation agencies will continue to scrutinize the delivery of healthcare in our country. The consumer demand for increased patient quality and safety will far outweigh any of the other issues mentioned previously. Shortages of staff, shortages of money, and other pressing issues will not take precedence over patient safety and quality, nor should they.

It is our responsibility as nursing leaders to look at these regulations and meet them to the best of our ability. As time goes on, there will be more and more of what we call "unfunded mandates." This means that the government and other accrediting bodies will put more regulations upon healthcare organizations. However, there will be no additional funding to help with compliance. So how does a nurse leader look at this and use creativity in the delivery of care and in dealing with other issues? As time goes on, we will be challenged continuously to look at new ways of delivering higher-quality and safer services.

Healthcare terminology

Competency in healthcare and medical terminology is required for any leadership position in healthcare. When it comes to the education of our leaders, we not only talk about healthcare terminology, but the terminology of healthcare in general. We have been called the profession of "alphabet soup," and we have an obligation to explain that alphabet soup to the general public, rather than using our own little euphemisms and shortcuts describing what is happening in healthcare.

Healthcare economics

How is healthcare intertwined with our economy? Why is it important for us to understand the economics of healthcare in the scheme of delivering care? If we do not understand the economics of healthcare and how it affects our society, we will be less able to be a leader in healthcare. The business of healthcare is increasingly important in our economy. Healthcare continues to be the largest component of our country's gross national product—currently around 18%. When reviewing open jobs, the two major areas of hiring in our economy right now are education and healthcare. Expenditures for healthcare continue to increase and will continue to increase over the next 10 to 20 years. A complete understanding of the economics of this and how it relates to our society is important as we think about new ways to deliver healthcare and the implementation of more efficient and better methodologies.

LEADERSHIP

TIP

Read journals and online news to stay on top of issues. Educate yourself so you can be a resource for your staff.

Technological research and advancement

Technology will continue to play an increasing role in the delivery of healthcare in our society and around the world. The understanding of what technology can do to make us more efficient in the delivery of care, better diagnostics, and better patient outcome is paramount for any healthcare leader. We must embrace technology and support its development, especially from a nursing perspective. Compared to other areas, there has been little technology invested in making nurses' jobs more efficient. Although we have computerized charting, robots, monitoring, and other technological efficiencies, nursing still could use further development in the area of the technological assistance in patient care.

Interaction and integration among healthcare sectors

How is healthcare coordinated and delivered throughout your region? Is there any coordination among providers? Do we as nursing leaders have a responsibility to assist in the development of this process? Nurses should take the lead in integrating healthcare across all environments. Nursing has been instrumental in moving the issue of access to healthcare forward, but the integration of services across the board has yet to occur in many places, and the idea of a national electronic medical record—or even a medical record that multiple providers would have access to at a central point—has yet to be developed to a level where they are useful in patient care. Increased collaboration and interaction among providers within a single healthcare entity is the nurse leader's job. Coordination of care on the nursing unit should fall to the nurses, so that efficiencies of care can be conducted without too much overlap and duplication of services. The nurse leader who takes this role will be a valued member of the healthcare organization.

Legislative issues

A significant component of knowledge of the healthcare environment is an awareness of what legislative issues are out there and being an advocate for the patient. Patient advocacy has always been part of a nurse's job. When institutions that I worked in hired people with the title of "patient advocate," I went to administration and said the nurses are the patient advocates; there is no need for anybody else to do this job. Over time, we have lost sight of the fact that nurses fill this role. Being a nursing leader, it is important to remember that it is one of our important roles, and that providing patient care and being an advocate for the correct patient procedures and plan of care is our mandate.

Managed care models

As leaders in healthcare, it is our duty to understand how our financial structure is put together through managed care models, structures, and environments (e.g., group physicians, staff models, independent practice associations, preferred provider organizations). What types of physician organizations and insurance groupings provide financial services to our patients? In some areas there may be one or two providers, but in larger metropolitan areas there may be many more. How does the structure of these organizations affect the care of patients in our charge? Issues such as length of stay, the ability to have an insurance company pay for certain diagnostic procedures, and what may or may not be provided to patients are all important facts that we need to know as healthcare leaders. As mentioned earlier, it is also important for us to be advocates for the patient under these circumstances where they might not be able to get what they need.

Staff interactions

Nursing leaders need to understand the interaction of all the staff within healthcare organizations, including nurses, physicians, and allied health professionals. Whose role is what and who is responsible for delivering what part of the care are important components of a nursing leader's perspective on management. A complete understanding of all of the roles within the nursing leader's practice environment will lead to better patient outcomes and quality of care, as well as better integration of services and efficiencies.

Never isolate any level of staff. Remember, it's all about relationships.

Organization and delivery of healthcare

Nursing leaders must understand how healthcare is delivered across the board. If you work in a large organization where healthcare is being delivered in acute care and ambulatory care settings, as well as long-term care, then you may have a rather good picture of how healthcare is delivered. But once we get outside of the larger organizations, healthcare can be delivered on many different levels, in many different places. In rural parts of our world, healthcare is delivered by itinerants who make it a point of delivering healthcare to those who cannot reach it. Overall, leaders in healthcare need to understand how healthcare is delivered in their area of practice.

Socioeconomic environment

You need to understand the socioeconomic environment in which the organization functions. Do you work in an organization that is in an inner city? Do you work in an organization that is an upper-middle-class neighborhood? How does the location and socioeconomic environment of your organization affect the care of the patient? A complete understanding of the environment in which the leader works and care is delivered is important to the effectiveness and efficiencies within that environment. There may be tremendous dichotomies between the patients that come to the organization based on socioeconomic factors.

Make it a point to know your demographics. An understanding of your patient community will allow you to make better decisions on their needs.

Information standards

A final key factor is the standards that are applicable to information integration and interoperability. How is information moved throughout your organization? Do you have systems that talk to each other? Do you have any systems at all? The integration of information is paramount to delivery of safe, quality patient care. More and more healthcare organizations are moving toward integrated records so that all healthcare providers understand and have access to what's happening with the patient. What standards within your organization govern information as it is passed around the organization? As a leader, you will be an information resource for the other people in your organization. Therefore, you should seek out the standards and processes that relate to information integration.

References

Healthcare Financial Management. January 2006 (60)1: 78.

Healthcare Leadership Alliance (2006). "HLA Competency Directory." Available at *www.healthcareleadershipalliance.org.*

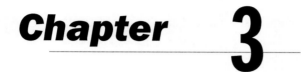

Chapter 3

COMPETENCIES FOR HEALTHCARE LEADERS: PROFESSIONALISM AND BUSINESS SKILLS

Learning objectives

After reading this section, the participant should be able to:

- Describe the benefits of maintaining high standards of professionalism
- Describe the business skill competencies essential for healthcare leaders
- Discuss strategies to improve competence in business skills

One of the key aspects of being a successful leader is being competent, doing a good job, and displaying a professional demeanor. This chapter discusses some aspects you need to master to develop your all-around competence.

Professionalism

Leaders who possess professionalism behave in accordance with ethical and professional standards, which include responsibilities to the patient and the communities served. Leaders have responsibilities to a service orientation and a commitment to lifelong learning and improvements.

Professionalism is something that you have likely been hearing about since basic education in nursing school. Unfortunately, sometimes we lose sight of what professionalism is as we advance through our careers. It is the responsibility of nursing leaders to role-model professionalism to the organization.

Benefits of professionalism

There are many aspects that make up professionalism, some of which are discussed in the following sections.

Organizational business and personal ethics: Above all, leaders must be ethical, both in their personal business and within their business operations. Ethical behavior is personal, and is learned at an early age. As a leader, it is always the right thing to take the "high road" in any questionable situation. Above other things, unethical behavior is intolerable for leaders.

Professional roles, responsibility, and accountability: Nursing leaders need to understand the professional roles of healthcare providers in the organization. The ability to understand other providers' responsibilities and what they are accountable for is something that will allow nursing leaders to better deliver the services necessary in their environment. It is their professional responsibility to be accountable, and leaders must also be accountable for the actions of their followers.

Professional norms and behaviors: Nursing leaders are responsible for knowing what professional norms and behaviors are required for those people who work for them. Additionally, we should also know what professional norms and behaviors are expected of all other healthcare providers with whom we interact. A leader's role involves maintaining professional accountability across the board.

Professional societies, memberships, standards, and codes of ethics: As leaders, we have a professional obligation to belong to membership organizations and societies that support our profession. Membership in these organizations is not the only requirement. We also need to participate in these organizations to understand and help shape their future. All professional organizations establish standards and codes of ethics for the profession, and it is a leader's responsibility to understand these standards, teach them to their staff, and enforce them.

Time and stress management techniques: If we cannot effectively manage our time and control our stress, then we cannot be effective leaders. Time management is one of the most important things that we can do as a leader. The demands that are placed on us on a regular basis always affect our priorities. Prioritization, time management, and controlling stress are important for maintaining our own health and development. Demands put on us by the people we lead continue to put pressure on our ability to handle all the needs that they have. Efficiency and effectiveness as a leader increases as the ability to manage our time improves.

Conflict-of-interest situations as defined by organizational bylaws, policies, and procedures: Conflict of interest is a serious problem for any leader. Most of what constitutes a conflict of interest is defined by your organization, but common sense should also help you identify conflicts of interest. It is important for you to read all conflict of interest policies and abide by them, as conflicts of interest can ruin your career.

Ethics committees' role, structure, and function: Every healthcare organization should have an ethics committee or some structure that handles ethical issues. As a leader in any healthcare organization, it is important to understand the role of the ethics committee, its function and structure, and what it deals with.

Patient rights and responsibilities: As a nursing leader, you are a patient advocate. Understanding patient rights and responsibilities is not only a role of the leader, but the role of everyone within the organization. As a leader, you should be sure that the entire staff knows the patient rights and responsibilities and respects them. It is also important as a leader to know when patients are not upholding their end of the responsibility. Healthcare is a shared experience between the patient and staff. Consequently, if patients do not uphold their responsibilities, leaders need to step in and interact with the patients. Therefore, it is important that leaders understand the responsibility of the patients and the staff in every healthcare environment.

Strategies to improve business skill competencies

Competent healthcare management leaders should be able to apply basic business principles, including organizational and analytical thinking, to the healthcare environment. The following key business skills are discussed in the remainder of this chapter:

- Financial management
- Human resources management
- Information management and technology
- Quality improvement
- Strategic planning and marketing

Financial management

In reviewing the necessary skills for financial management, some may be unfamiliar to you. If you have not received education in a business or administrative capacity, some of these terms and principles may be very new to you. However, as a developing leader, you need to understand these financial terms. As discussed earlier, the clinical staff and leadership of the institution must be able to understand its financial components in order to compete on a level playing field.

LEADERSHIP

TIP

Make it your business to learn the nuances of the finance office. You need to speak their language to be deemed competent.

Cost accounting: The practice of cost accounting is the analysis of what things actually cost. For example, we may charge $1,000 for an MRI, but if we broke down the actual costs of administering an MRI, we may find that it only costs us $300. Therefore, our profit margins are $700. Cost accounting allows us to ascertain what things actually cost us, so that we can charge an appropriate fee for something.

Financial analysis: This includes ratio analysis, cost-benefit analysis, cost-effectiveness analysis, vertical analysis, and horizontal analysis. Although most of us were not trained as accountants, it is important to understand the purpose of these analyses. The information provided by these analyses will allow us to understand whether programs can be efficient and make money while providing a necessary service.

Cost-effectiveness and cost-benefit analyses, although similar in terminology, are actually different approaches. In cost-effectiveness, we look at whether a certain program is providing what we need and whether it is cost-effective. Cost-benefit analysis weighs not only the financial component, but also whether the services are necessary. This includes looking at margins and whether the program is a valued service for the organization. Even though the financial margin may be slim, we may decide to use the program because it provides a benefit to our organization.

Financial planning methodologies: This includes strategic planning, strategic financial planning, operational planning, budgeting, and capital budgeting. When performing financial analyses it is important to understand the strategic planning process from both an organizationwide structure and financial planning structure perspective. Budgeting and capital budgeting are the most elementary financial processes that nurse leaders need to understand. Budgeting is the simple process of putting together the amount of financial resources necessary to run the operation, which is sometimes restricted by the amount of income that is allowed to a unit. The skills of creating a budget are outside the scope of this book.

Financial statements: The ability to read and interpret the financial statements for your unit and for the entire organization is a necessary skill for leaders. Without the knowledge of the financial operations within your organization, you cannot run it efficiently or understand the possibilities for program expansion or retraction. Financial statements will give you the entire financial picture of the unit or your organization. Financial statements can be very simple or very complicated, depending on the size of operations that you support. It is important for you to educate yourself in this area.

LEADERSHIP

TIP

This is a good area to engage in extra study. There are many excellent resources on the market that can increase your knowledge and your self-confidence.

Outcome measures and management: This includes return on investment (ROI), cost-effectiveness analyses, cash flow analysis, and testing. If you are looking to start a new program within your organization, it is important to understand what your ROI will be. For example, if we invested $1,000 into a program and the program actually costs us $1,200 to run, then our ROI would be −$200. Obviously, you would not want to start or maintain this program.

Cash flow analysis is the most important analysis of any organization. Leaders and organizations should know how many days of cash there are on hand in the bank. In other words, if no money came into the organization over the next month or week or day, how many days will the organization be able to sustain itself before it goes broke? An appropriate analogy is if you had lost your job and needed to know how many days you could last on the money that you have in your bank. When interviewing for a leadership role, it is important to ask the question of how many days of cash the organization has on hand. The more days it has, the better off it is financially.

It is important to remember two rules when discussing cash. The first rule is that "cash is king," and the second is that "he who controls the gold makes the rules." If leaders are involved in creating or allocating the cash flow, then their position within the organization becomes all the more important and powerful.

Fundamental productivity measures: This includes hours per patient day, cost per patient day, units of service per man-hour, or per member per month. Productivity measures in nursing are extremely important. Every nursing leader knows that the largest budget in any healthcare institution, hospital, or ambulatory care center is the cost of nursing care. Therefore, it is important that we have productivity measures to be sure that the budget is maintained, appropriate patient care is given, and we have enough financial resources to provide safe, quality care.

There are many schools of thought on measuring nursing productivity, but if we focus on the basics, the hour per patient day method is still the most appropriate. It is easy to monitor and inexpensive to analyze and set; it does not change with the census; and it is a solid benchmark from which to justify budgetary expenditures within nursing. The right sizing of a nursing budget is a very important measure for the administration of any healthcare organization, and setting the budget on hours per patient day is one way to measure consistency from shift to shift and day to day. The cost per patient day on a unit is another way to measure productivity and efficiency. By comparing hours per patient day and the cost per patient day, we can evaluate whether our unit is financially solvent. Of course, other measures contribute to the financial solvency of any particular unit, but if we know what it costs to deliver patient care and we know what it costs per hour of patient care delivery, then we will know whether we are cost-effective.

Operating budget principles: This includes fixed versus flexible and zero-based. Every organization has its own budgeting principles. If you are already involved in the budgeting process of your organization, then you will know what type of budgets you use on an annual basis. Once again, the budgeting process is an education in itself, and it is useful to read and educate yourself further on this process. However, note that understanding the principles of budget construction is one of the fundamental jobs of a manager, and to be a good leader within the organization, you need to have very good budgeting skills and a comprehensive understanding of financial systems.

Revenue cycle and accounts receivable management processes: Revenue cycle and accounts receivable are primary operations within the organization. An understanding of the revenue cycle in your organization, the time it takes to collect money, the time it takes to bill clients, and how that money comes in and is spent are important in understanding the cash flow of the organization. Organizations that have slow payers will have what is known as a significant number of "days in accounts receivable." The longer the days in accounts receivable, the harder it is to collect money. Once again, this financial management skill is one that you must investigate further, but it is outside the scope of this book.

Human resource management

For leaders in any healthcare organization, one of the areas of focus is human resources. We are a human resource–intensive industry, where as much as 75% of any healthcare organization's budget may be related to expenditures on human resources. Developing the next generation of leaders in an organization is a critical human resource competency. Future leaders should be chosen because they are qualified to move into leadership roles, not just because they have succeeded in their current role. As a leader, or someone who is trying to develop new leaders, your human resource and interpersonal skills are going to be your most important competence.

To be effective in human resource management, you need to have knowledge of the following skills and issues.

Compensation and benefits: An understanding of how your employees are compensated and what benefits they will receive is important not only in the recruiting process but also in retention of your employees. In today's nursing shortage, retention of our best and brightest is one of the most important things a leader can do. Turnover of our best and brightest will cost the organization a significant amount of money. To that end, it is also important to compensate employees appropriately and provide them with benefits that will allow them to feel comfortable in a position and stay in the organization. In most cases it is not up to nursing leadership to decide what the salary package will be, but rather to understand it and be able to discuss it with employees as necessary.

Employee satisfaction measurement and improvement techniques: How do we know our employees are satisfied? How do we know whether our employees are productive and improving on an annual basis? Employee satisfaction is measured annually by many organizations. It is a good measure of whether the people who work in the organization are happy and, if they are not, a good way to identify the reasons why.

Performance improvement should happen on a continuous basis, not just at the end of the year. Employee performance improvement is something that we can use to find new leaders and people who want to advance within our organizations. Leaders are constantly helping their employees improve their performance and work on skills they need to move onto other positions within the organization.

LEADERSHIP

TIP

Begin to identify who could be you. If you didn't come back tomorrow, who would take your job? Would you be happy with that? If not, develop your successor.

Motivational techniques: All leaders are motivators. A distinguishing quality of a leader is one who can motivate people toward a common goal. But motivational skills take practice. Not everyone can be a good motivator, but anyone who aspires to be a leader needs to develop motivational skills to reach the goals necessary for success.

Organizational policies and procedures and their functions: All organizational leaders need to be able to interpret policy and procedures for their employees. They do not necessarily have to memorize the entire 400-page policy book, but a working knowledge of how to interpret what policies and procedures are doing for them and the organization is an important leadership skill.

Human resources laws and regulations: This includes wages, the Family Medical Leave Act, the Equal Employment Opportunity Commission, the Employee Retirement Income Security Act, and Workers' Compensation. As a nursing leader, it is important to understand where to find resources for information on the human resource laws and regulations in your organization. A basic working knowledge of all of them is very important, but it is not your role as a nursing leader or manager to understand all of the idiosyncrasies of all of these laws.

 A Practical Guide to Leadership Development

As a nursing leader, you should be able to use your human resource contacts for help when you encounter an issue in one of these areas.

LEADERSHIP

TIP

Your human resource professionals are one of your best resources for issues and problems. Use them extensively. Remember, it's all about relationships.

Staffing methodologies and productivity management: This includes acuity-based staffing, flexible staffing, and fixed staffing. When it comes to human resource management, this is the big stuff. Early on as a nurse leader, you have to learn that there are two things that you do not mess with: your employees' time and money. As nursing leaders, staffing and scheduling are the most important things that you are going to do for your employees. Trying to please all the people all the time is not going to happen, so you must bring out your best leadership skills to look at things from a fair and equitable basis and deal with all of the conflicts that may occur, especially around the time of holiday scheduling.

However, an effective and efficient staffing plan is the key to good financial management. When there is a need to cut the budget or eliminate inefficiencies, many organizations look to the nursing department because it is the largest component of human resource dollars. If you have a good staffing, scheduling, and monitoring plan in place, it will be difficult to find inefficiencies or a way to cut any positions, because you are delivering the right amount of care, by the right provider, to the right patient, at the right time, for the right money. Maintaining efficient schedules is also a very good employee satisfier.

LEADERSHIP

TIP

Personnel costs are the highest cost in the organization. Know how to develop and manage an efficient staffing plan. There are many resources that you can refer to that will help you develop this skill.

Information management and technology

Use of information and technology are more and more synonymous every day. As technology enters the workplace, the exchange and use of information becomes easier. As leaders in an organization, we must embrace technology and the use of information in providing safe, efficient, and quality patient care. As leaders, we also need to continuously think about improving the way information is handled in an organization and what we can do to improve the utilization of the information that technology provides. As leaders in any organization, there are many areas where technology is improving and gaining greater usage, and there is information that pertains specifically to nursing.

Applications software: Spreadsheets, e-mail, word processing, and database applications are the most fundamental software for you to work with. As nursing leaders, you must be able to use these software packages to increase efficiency and be able to participate on a high level. Few people today do not use e-mail, but plenty of people do not use spreadsheets and databases. If you know you have a learning deficit in these particular areas, then you must seek out education to ensure that you are playing on the same field as everybody else.

LEADERSHIP

TIP

If you know how to use spreadsheets, your life will be a lot easier and you will be able to do your analysis without relying on anyone else.

Characteristics of administrative systems/programs: This includes financial, scheduling, online purchasing, productivity, and human resources. Within every organization, there are administrative systems and programs that support the infrastructure and the backbone of the organization. Financial systems are in place to maintain the financial solvency of the organization. They may also be in place for you to develop and monitor your budget and see other financial data necessary for the development of programs. Many organizations today use scheduling software that helps them maintain balanced schedules and provide human resource data important to the nursing department's operation. Many organizations also use online purchasing software that allows you to log onto your personal computer and select the items that you want to order, which will then be delivered directly to your unit within a selected time. Productivity software can fall into the financial or human resource department, depending on what type of productivity you are looking at. On the human resource side, this data includes overtime, sick time, hours per patient day, and so on, which can help improve productivity.

Characteristics of clinical systems/programs: This includes electronic medical records, medical decision support, and diagnostic information systems. There are great differences in the clinical systems at various organizations. Some have electronic medical records, others have medical decision support, and the rest have diagnostic information systems. In the early

A Practical Guide to Leadership Development

development of clinical information systems, the prime motivation was to collect information in order to get accurate billing. In today's clinical information systems, it is directed toward getting accurate and efficient clinical information for diagnostic purposes. We are still very much in the early stages of technology implementation on the clinical system side of healthcare. Over the next five years, we will see a significant increase in the use of technology to assist us in the delivery of clinical services.

Data analysis: Data analysis includes the manipulation of, understanding of, and ability to explain data. With the advent of powerful desktop computing, we can now do significant data analysis right at our desktop. Twenty-five years ago, the use of mainframes was the primary way to do statistical analysis. Today there are programs that do not require any significant statistical knowledge to crunch data. By storing data in spreadsheets, we can also manipulate data in any way we need in order to understand what it reports and use it as a powerful tool for making effective clinical and administrative decisions.

Electronic education and information resources: Education has now entered the technological age with the advent of learning management systems and online educational programs. As time progresses, we will also see increased use of technology for long-distance meetings, instant learning resources, bedside information at the touch of a button, and hand-held devices that provide more information than can be held in 25 textbooks. As leaders, we know it is important to provide education for all followers. If we cannot provide it, then we must know which resources will. An increasingly intelligent workforce is the best way to deliver better, safer patient care.

Health informatics: This includes coding, communication standards, and data standards. To be effective and efficient, healthcare systems need to be able to "talk" to each other and communicate between systems, with an even exchange of data and information. As health informatics continues to progress, the codes and communication language of the systems will become more and more compatible, allowing communication across all platforms. A basic understanding of health informatics is important to developing nurse leaders.

Information technology planning and implementation: As nursing becomes more and more involved in the implementation of technology throughout healthcare organizations, a working knowledge of the larger picture of information technology is necessary in order to be successful. Over the next five years nursing will play a greater role in the implementation of technology throughout an organization. The advent of electronic medical records and more tools to make nursing more efficient will be at the forefront of changes in healthcare. The ability to work with the information technology department in system selection, criteria, and review will also be an important competency for nursing leaders.

LEADERSHIP TIP Make it a point to understand technology to the best of your ability. Take classes, learn it on your own, read, and so on. Knowing technology applications will help you be a better leader as you find solutions to improve efficiency and develop better clinical outcomes.

Principles of database and file management: A basic understanding of how technology works, how databases are constructed, and how to mine the data from these databases will become an important skill for nursing leaders in the future. The more you know about databases and file management, the more valuable you will be to any organization. Not only will you be valuable to the organization, but also to the people who work for you and the patients.

Quality improvement

There are more and more demands on healthcare systems for improving quality. Some payment organizations are moving to pay for performance, and if your organization does not have good quality outcomes, it will not get paid for certain cases. With such a connection between quality and financial survival, it is imperative that nursing leaders understand, promote, practice, and develop quality management techniques.

Nurse leaders need to have competency and knowledge of the following areas of quality improvement.

Clinical pathways and disease management: Nursing leaders should take the lead in using clinical pathways in the management of disease. Disease management is a concept that has been around for many years, but has not taken off because it would need significant buy-in from the entire healthcare community. Disease management is a process that happens both in and out of acute care settings, with the primary goal of keeping people with chronic diseases out of acute care institutions. Clinical pathways have been shown to improve efficiencies and care within organizations, but they are not good for every case. As we know, today many patients come into our institutions with comorbidities, which mean patients move off a clinical pathway because of other complications. Clinical pathways cannot account for every clinical problem that arises. Therefore, when it comes to implementation, there are mixed opinions about the use of clinical pathways.

Customer satisfaction principles and tools: These were discussed earlier on in the relationship management section.

Data collection, measurement, and analysis tools and techniques: This includes root cause analysis, process analysis, and workflows. Educated decisions are the only decisions we should be making when it comes to quality outcomes. With the availability of technology and software packages that can easily analyze data, there is no excuse for failing to measure and analyze data that we collect on our patients. Leaders are responsible for the quality outcomes of the patients, and so they should work with and through their employees to ensure positive patient outcomes in the organization. Once again, financial reimbursement will be based on quality outcomes in the near future—this is happening in some organizations right now. This particular plan is known as "pay for performance," and if your performance is poor, you will not get paid. The nurse leader is on the front line when it comes to quality performance. As a patient advocate, and in some cases the coordinator of care, the nurse leader works with other healthcare providers in ensuring quality outcomes for the patient.

National quality initiatives including patient safety: As a healthcare leader, you are responsible and accountable for knowing what the national quality initiatives are, as well as the patient safety initiatives for your organization. Patient safety initiatives should not be told to us and handed down from above, but should be issues that we inherently know about. Recommendations and guidelines from professional organizations and governmental agencies should be followed closely, to ensure the best outcome and safest environment for the patient.

Patient communication systems: How do we communicate with and through our patients? Communication systems range from how we give patient reports to electronic systems that allow us to communicate directly with the patient from anywhere in the organization. Communication systems are a necessary part of daily patient care management. "System" in this case does not necessarily mean an electronic system, but rather a methodology for communicating effectively with the patient population in your area of responsibility.

Quality improvement theories and frameworks: Quality improvement processes are essentially research projects that should use evidence as a basis for improving patient care. The literature has presented us with numerous methods for putting quality assurance and improvement plans in effect. Later in this book, we will discuss the PDCA methodology of performance improvement. Leaders need to have competency in this area because it is one of the core competencies of nursing leadership, and an ability to look at the evidence of why or why not something is happening is key. If there are positive outcomes with certain procedures, it is just as important to find the reasons behind this as it is to find out why things may not be happening because of poor process. The establishment of evidence-based practice is beginning to transform the way we deliver care. If a leader is doing research in an organization, it is important to document that research and find out whether the changes put into place are making any difference in the outcome of patient care. The simple fact that there is evidence supporting or negating a certain process helps us to move toward better quality outcomes.

Quality planning and management: As just mentioned, the ability to plan for new quality studies and the ability to manage the quality of the unit are essential traits of a leader. Planning for quality outcomes on the unit involves the utilization of the staff, evidence, and other healthcare professionals to decide whether certain procedures or practices are effective in maintaining quality patient outcomes. Nursing's role in most organizations is the provision of quality care. With the advent of technology, the ability to almost instantaneously look up evidence related to a certain procedure should allow us to provide better quality care in the years to come as we get used to using it.

Training and certification: All good leaders educate and develop their staff. In the realm of quality management, it is important that staff understand the process of improving care in certain situations. By gathering data, analyzing the data, and providing education and training, leaders can improve the quality outcome of our patients significantly. There is now a certification exam in quality management, and numerous other continuing education programs can be found regarding this subject.

Utilization review and management regulations: Appropriate utilization of health resources is a nursing leader's role. Misuse of scarce resources costs not only the organization money, but the consumers as well. As the cost of healthcare continues to rise, the utilization of appropriate resources necessary to maintain health and well-being should be the leader's focus. Health maintenance organizations and other insurance providers keep healthcare costs for their members down by continuously monitoring the utilization of services and hospitalization of their membership. As nursing leaders, it is important that we also review the utilization of these resources, because ultimately misuse will make it impossible for us to provide the necessary care to people who might really need it.

Strategic planning and marketing

As the needs and demands of the healthcare system change, we must constantly plan and change with it. One necessary skill for the nurse leader is the ability to strategically plan and market services. It begins with the vision and goals that leaders set for organizations. But goals and visions cannot be set in a vacuum; there must be a process for making them goal-oriented and realistic. This process is strategic planning. Whether we are planning a new service, putting a business plan together, developing crisis and disaster planning, or planning for healthcare system services, leaders need to understand the process and how to make it effective and efficient.

There are numerous competencies nurse leaders need for strategic planning and marketing purposes.

Business plan development and implementation processes: If leaders are responsible for setting the vision, direction, goals, and objectives of the organization, then the process of business planning is paramount to their success. Business plan development and implementation are necessary if a new service is going into a unit, if there is going to be a downsizing of the service in the unit, or if you want to plan for a service that is in demand in your particular area. Business planning is both a science and an art. It is a science because it is based on financial data, and an art because it requires some guesswork in forecasting the future.

Business planning including business case and exit strategy development: How do you develop a business case for something new? Gone are the days when we can just say, "I think we need to put something in place because . . . " A business case is a much better way to put something into action. Exit strategies are just the opposite. For example, if we have been running a dialysis unit in our organization for many years, and now we decide we are going to close that service, how do we exit that business without hurting anybody financially, clinically, or otherwise?

Crisis and disaster planning: In today's unsettled world, crisis and disaster planning are necessary competencies for every leader in every organization. The development of disaster and contingency operation plans—from small blackouts or electrical outages to large acts of terrorism—is a skill of which all leaders should have a working knowledge. Many of these skills can be obtained by logging onto the Federal Emergency Management Agency (FEMA) Web site and looking for some of the free education programs. There is also a information in the literature on how to handle crises and disaster issues.

Healthcare system services: When looking at strategic planning, it is important to note the needs of the community, the other providers that are meeting those needs, and where there is a need to provide an additional service. Identifying needed services is part of the strategic planning process. Once those services are in place, then it becomes increasingly necessary to market those services so that the business case for their survival is positive.

Additional competencies

Many of the skills necessary to lead can be found in the competencies listed in this chapter. In order to develop effective leaders, healthcare organizations must know what specific competencies are required. This chapter listed many competencies that leaders need to have to make organizations and themselves successful. When developing leaders, there are basic core competencies and then there are advanced competencies. The following chapters discuss in detail some of the core competencies necessary to be a leader and develop new leadership on your units. Management today has many complex challenges and opportunities that require all healthcare executives to have extraordinary skill sets. The question today is how do we know that leaders have them? If they don't have them, how do we develop those skills?

Unfortunately, nursing seems to lack a surge in leadership and leadership development. But the future needs good, competent, visionary leaders. It is a leader's job to assess and enhance the leadership skills of staff members who might move into a leadership role. It is also a leader's responsibility to assess the capabilities of potential new hires from outside the organization and decide whether they have the ability to move into leadership. If they do, put them on the fast track. It is a responsibility of the academic environment to ensure that students of healthcare management, nursing administration, and other leadership programs are trained to fulfill specific leadership competencies while allowing their future employers to fulfill their missions. True leaders are always optimistic; the glass is always half full, and never half empty, and good leaders will get you to see it the same way. Leaders are motivators who are able to build relationships, collaborate, and put the resources together in order to achieve goals to make their organization great.

Further resources

A complete list of competencies for healthcare management can be found at *www.healthcareleadershipalliance.org*. The Healthcare Leadership Alliance comprises the nation's premier professional societies, representing more than 100,000 members across the healthcare management disciplines. It includes the following organizations:

- American College of Healthcare Executives (ACHE)

- American Organization of Nurse Executives (AONE)

- Healthcare Financial Management Association (HFMA)

- Healthcare Information and Management Systems Society (HIMSS)

- Medical Group Management Association (MGMA) and its certification body, the American College of Medical Practice Executives (ACMPE)

Chapter 4

SYSTEMS THINKING:
BIG THINKING FOR LOCAL SUCCESS

Learning objectives

After reading this section, the participant should be able to:

- Explain the concept of systems thinking
- Discuss how healthcare leaders can use systems thinking to improve their organizations

What is systems thinking?

Systems thinking is a framework of thought that helps people deal with complex situations and concepts in a holistic way. To understand systems thinking, we must first understand what a system is. Reviewing a variety of resources, a system can be defined as an entity that maintains its existence and functions as a whole through the interaction and collaboration of its parts. Systems thinking looks at the entire system as a whole, including its parts and the connections and interactions between the parts. When you look at the pattern that connects the parts rather than simply the parts themselves, you will see that the pattern drives the behavior of the system. It has been said that you can then make predictions about the system without knowing all the parts in detail.

Systems thinking provides a set of ideas, tools, and methods for engaging with and improving complex situations, created by human activity, where everything seems to be connected to everything else. Examples include implementing organizational change, dealing with difficult relationships, and making decisions about environmental issues.

LEADERSHIP

TIP

Think of your environment as a system: It is complex and has many intricacies. Step back and take a look from the outside: It will be different.

Why is systems thinking so important? Simply put, we are living in a world of systems. The natural environment is a huge complex system; towns and cities where we live are systems; and the organizations where we work are systems. We also have systems such as computers and cars, and we can talk about political systems and economic systems.

Each of these systems works as a complete functioning whole combining many similar parts. Systems can be simple or complex. If we look at the human body we find numerous systems that function together to create the whole. We can study these in isolation, or we can study the human body as a whole. We also look at systems thinking as thinking in circles, rather than in straight lines. All parts and services are connected directly or indirectly, where a change in one part will have a ripple effect to all other parts of the system. This changes all the other parts, and after the cycle is completed, the influence of what happens comes back to the original part in some modified way. Creating this loop is called "feedback."

Example of systems thinking

In healthcare, one of the most obvious feedback loops we have is in our quality management systems, and you may be surprised to learn that the quality management process is a systems thinking tool. When we look at root cause analysis, or systems such as Plan, Do, Check, and Act (PDCA), we have created feedback loops to give us information that we need to do our jobs on an everyday basis. This is just one example of the importance of systems thinking.

A Practical Guide to Leadership Development

LEADERSHIP

TIP

Review a recent quality issue in your area and see if you can make a decision on cause without all the facts. When you do, you have entered into the systems thinking process.

Systems thinking and your organization

Systems thinking has also been defined as a way for understanding change, uncertainty, and complexity, and for creating harmony of thoughts and actions. Every good manager and leader must develop systems thinking, as it is increasingly necessary to understand the interdependence within our healthcare system and its complexity. Need for leadership and decision-making at all levels of work, shared visions, and alignment with the individual mission, vision, and values of the organization requires systems thinking. Systems thinking is something that can also be used outside of the healthcare environment. Our society and world are complex, and systems thinking helps us deal with all problems—not just in our work environment, but in our private lives as well.

Other examples of systems theories

Some better-known examples of systems theories include the following:

1. Robert Blake and Jane Mouton (1964) developed a theory known as the "Managerial Grid." It is based on two variables: focus on task and focus on relationships. The grid includes five possible leadership styles based on concern for task or concern for people. Using a specially designed testing instrument, people can be assigned a numerical score depicting their concern for each variable. Numerical indications, such as 9,1 or 9,9 or 1,9 or 1,1 or 5,5 can then be plotted on the grid using horizontal and vertical axes. Although Blake and Mouton's work is also often classified as a leadership theory, it is typical of the specially designed analysis and instruments of the systems theorists.

2. Victor Vroom (2002) studied the motivational and decision-making processes and developed what has come to be known as expectancy theory (also known as equity theory as developed by Homans and other social psychologists). This approach attempts to measure the degree of desire to perform a behavior rather than the need to perform a behavior. Motivation strength is calculated by multiplying the

perceived value of the result of performing a behavior by the perceived probability that the result will materialize. The idea that workers are driven by complex internal processes of motivation is sometimes known as *expectancy theory*.

3. Fred Fiedler (1967) devised a questionnaire called the "Least Preferred Coworker (LPC) Scale," which can be used by management in various ways, but most importantly in this context to find out what integrates or interrelates the human subsystem. Fiedler believed in situational leadership, that some personality attributes contribute to effective leadership in some situations but not in others. The idea that there is no single best approach to leadership is sometimes known as *contingency theory*.

Nine principles of systems

Dr. Kambiz Maani (2002) set out nine principles of systems:

1. Cause and effect are often not close in time and space. Quick results may be misleading. The time between decisions and results may be much longer than expected and may show itself in a very different place.

2. Today's problems are often caused by yesterday's solutions (linked to the first principle).

3. All actions have feedback. There is a false expectation that the world is linear. Actions can produce results that impact back on action taken.

4. There is often talk of either "this" or "that," but there is likely to be a number of issues in between (rather than either/or). The tendency to accept one and reject the others is shallow and ignores multiple possibilities.

5. Results are not proportional to effort. We expect them to be proportional to effort because we expect the world to be linear.

6. We contribute to our own problems through our assumptions, values, beliefs, and unintended consequences of our actions. The system itself generates a lot of its own problems.

7. A system is as good as its weakest link—there is often a focus on "star perform-ance" at the expense of ignoring the weaker parts.

8. There is more than what we can "see." Soft measures, such as staff morale, commit-ment, and respect for leadership, are powerful indicators of performance.

9. The structure of systems determines its behavior—there is a lot of interest in changing behavior, but this will not happen if attention is not paid to the structure driving the change.

Paramount to this entire discussion is the fact that the whole is made up of parts. In today's healthcare environment, we must remember that every service unit is looked at as part of a larger system that will "drill down" to the direction that the unit has to take in its relationship to other parts of the organization. Every unit in the institution is required to ensure that it fits well within the activities of other units, or its value to the system as a whole is diminished. Systems theory will tell us that the working relationships between the components of the system are just as important as the work of any one of its individual components. One of the more common problems within healthcare organizations is that the people who work in individual units are focused and directed only on the work of those individual units and their intentions for positive outcomes within it. Because they live and work within that unit, they forget that whatever they do has broad ramifications to the organization as a whole.

Leaders in healthcare organizations must keep focused on the organization's broader purpose, mission, vision, and values. The leader must ensure that there is a fit between the activities of those at the point of service and the overall work of the organization. This takes a considerable amount of work because it is very difficult to focus outside of an individual unit when there are so many issues affecting it on a daily basis. If leaders spend every day at the point of service and get caught up in the day-to-day activities, they ultimately forget what the larger goals of the organization are and sometimes have difficulty integrating that unit into the overall system.

Impact of systems thinking on organizational change

Traditional approaches to organizational management have emphasized the analysis of individual problems and incremental change, but this will no longer suffice as companies continue to experience complex changes. It is becoming increasingly more difficult to see the consequences of our decisions and to learn from experience. Systems thinking has given companies a tool with which they can better cope with this constant change. It allows individuals to see processes over time and to break away from the assumptions that have prevented lasting results. Systems thinking is now being used in combination with other organizational change strategies (Gardner and Demello 1993).

Systems vs. institutions

To this point, we have been discussing systems and institutions as if they were one and the same. They are not. An institution's focus is on most of the work being done in silos in a vertical pattern, where the focus on the process of getting the work done sometimes creates clear separations between what is happening in that particular area and others within the organization. At the point of care, the focus is usually on productivity and positive outcomes. In most organizations, if we look at the organizational chart, we will find a vertical pyramid. This vertical pyramid tells us a lot about the organization and its function and reporting mechanisms. Systems focus on a strong alignment of everyone involved in the organization, are outcomes driven, and have the feedback loop in a circular structure that was discussed earlier in this chapter.

Many problems arise in organizations because of the inability of leaders to think and act laterally as well as vertically. Leaders and managers must be able to see the whole and understand how the parts function together. Creating a whole structure of the system will enable leaders to see and act within a systems approach and keep in touch with the demands of the whole while simultaneously focusing on positive outcomes of the local unit. A major function of today's healthcare manager is to build relationships with other clinical departments and other departments within the organization and to try to break down the boundaries between them, in order to create a continuum of care by better integration of all of the services provided. As we move forward in this direction, the comprehensiveness of a healthcare system will begin to emerge and take the structure of a system. With today's increasing technology, it is very possible to do this and eliminate the boundaries between clinical services to provide a better system of care.

Characteristics of effective systems

Effective systems have no more structure than is absolutely necessary for them to function. When there is too much structure, resources and work tend to stray away from the actual point of delivery. The more structure in a system, the more likely the system will support the structure rather than the service that it delivers, the more money the structure will cost the system, and the fewer the resources the system will have available. Therefore, the system will be less able to thrive and fulfill its purpose.

Within systems, everything operates from the center out. Most systems are organic in shape and design, usually in the form of a circle. This is because systems are more about relationships and the interaction of those relationships than anything else. Systems are fluid and dynamic, and entail interactions and relationships in a continuous interplay that results in fulfilling the mission of that particular system. All activities of the system must work together to help those systems adapt to changes, meet goals, and thrive.

The leader's role is to see to it that the purpose of the system and the needs of the patients are congruent and everything that the system does is directed toward meeting those needs in an appropriate manner.

The majority of conflicts within a system take place at the point of service. If the processes at a point of service are not structured to be a good fit with the system, the system will begin to break down. Most work done by leaders of systems today involves building relationships that will last and keeping the system intact and on course. Leaders seek congruence between purpose of the system and the work of the people in it; in doing this, leaders constantly face the challenge of the conflict between personal and system agendas. Good leaders must realize that the system's survival depends on the relationship between good structure and good process. Good leaders also focus on the system's flexibility and its ability to adapt quickly to changes in its environment. Doing this usually requires revision of the structure as the system grows, in order to position the system so it better serves its patient population. Leaders must also constantly monitor the system, and its structures and purposes, to ensure that the work processes are continuing to meet the needs of the patient population. The structure of the system should never be an obstacle to delivering what the system is supposed to.

Improving healthcare systems

Let's take a broader view of systems thinking within the healthcare environment. When looking at patient safety, we can no longer place blame just on human error. Improving patient safety today takes a more effective focus on human factors, engineering, and the systems within which healthcare professionals work. We know that systems thinking does not come naturally to us. We have been educated to recognize our personal responsibilities to master knowledge and skills and acquire wisdom that enables us to do our job, which is to assist the sick, vulnerable, and dependent. It has been said that a system is perfectly designed to produce the output data it produces; or, conversely, whatever output we get from a system is what the system is designed to produce.

As healthcare leaders, we are challenged to learn more about how to apply systems thinking to healthcare, through answering questions such as: Where are the micro and macro systems in healthcare? How can their performance be measured? How do they interact? What are the vulnerabilities and strengths? What are the strengths and weaknesses of each component that comprises the system? How can those strengths and weaknesses compensate for each other within the larger system? How can the functions of each component be optimized so results of the system can be maximized? How can we identify and monitor for unintended consequences, and how do we intervene to prevent harm coming from these? By asking ourselves these questions and looking at the larger picture of healthcare—not just within our organization, but from a global perspective—we as leaders in healthcare will be able to help set policy and agenda going forward.

Complex adaptive systems

Practitioners and organizations today are taking theories from the new sciences of complexity. These sciences are sometimes called chaotic, self organizing, nonlinear, complex adaptive, or emergent. These sciences give voice to institutions and the experiences of people who work competently to support change and human systems. One of the major roles of a leader and manager is to be a change agent, and in today's environment of complexity, this becomes increasingly more difficult. Therefore, it is important to understand what a complex adaptive system is, because these systems represent today's healthcare environment.

A complex adaptive system (CAS) is a collection of semiautonomous agents interacting in unpredictable ways and generating systemwide patterns over time. Examples of complex adaptive systems include the stock market, social insect and ant colonies, the biosphere and the ecosystem, the brain and the immune system, the cell and the developing embryo, manufacturing businesses, and any human social group–based endeavor in a cultural and social system, such as political parties or communities. The team is a good example of a CAS in human systems. Team members are agents, and each has a unique perspective and unique skills and interests. Through a variety of means, such as meetings, e-mails, and informal chats, the agents interact, and over time the team generates patterns of group behavior that can be observed in its work, the personal relationships between the members, and the members' individual growth and development. Sometimes the patterns are highly productive, and sometimes they are not, but the patterns will be identified as the behavior of the team apart from the contributions of individuals. Have you ever heard someone say that they would never work on a unit because it had a bad reputation, or the people were not very functional? This would be the outcome of that team behavior, not a reflection of the individuals. No unit has all "bad apples."

Most complex adaptive systems demonstrate similar behavior, regardless of the nature of the agents or the context of their engagements. Pascale, Millemann, and Gioja (2000) identified some of these characteristic behaviors:

Self-organization: The pattern of the whole emerges from the internal dynamics and operations of the system. It is not imposed from outside. Organizational culture, for example, emerges from the complex interactions of the people within the system, not from the outside or from a management decree.

Sensitive dependence on initial conditions: Very small changes can generate enormous effects. Sometimes this is called the "butterfly effect." This metaphor derives from the flap of a single butterfly wing that can change systemic patterns in parts of the system that are remote in space or in time. Rumors are a great example of the butterfly effect in an organization. The comment overheard in a lunch room can mushroom into a crisis of confidence or action.

Dynamism: A CAS is always in motion. You cannot judge the system's emerging existence by taking a single snapshot of the agents at any point in time. Even when a CAS appears to be in a stable state, its internal interactions tend to emerge over time. This is why when we are trying to evaluate the work of nurses, we cannot do it in a short period of time, such as one shift or even one week. Snapshots do not tell the story.

Nonlinear causality: In these highly interdependent systems, one thing causes and is simultaneously caused by something else. Trust is a good example of nonlinear causality in human system dynamics. You behave in such a way that I trust you, and I trust you because you behave in that way. This causal circle relationship makes it quite difficult to see which comes first, the behavior or the trust.

Fractal structures: Similar patterns are repeated at various levels and parts of a complex system. Repetition gives coherence to the whole, like the geometrical patterns of fractals or biological patterns of broccoli, where the part is a miniature version of the whole. Competitive individuals exist in competitive teams. Competitive teams emerge in competitive organizations. Competitive organizations thrive in competitive industries and economies. Because of this replicated structure, different levels of organizing individual teams or other organizations exhibit similar patterns and can be affected by similar interventions.

Path dependency: Each complex system is unique and therefore has a complex combination of patterns that emerge from a unique history. For each system, the future emerges out of the complex dynamics of the current moment. In this way, history is of major significance to the dynamics of human systems. Patterns of the present will be understood in terms of the dynamics of the past, although they were not predetermined by this. For example, an organization may have a vision, but its ability to make the vision a reality lies in its current capacity as patterns of performance that emerged in the past.

Managing in a complex adaptive system

When trying to manage in a CAS, you need to acknowledge the natural dynamics of the system, explore them, and work in concert and collaboration with them. Your path to solutions may be unpredictable, but your outcomes usually will be productive and satisfying to you, your staff, and the organization.

You can function effectively within the system by using multiple tools and approaches when trying to interact with the system. As stated earlier, because of the complexity and changing roles of the system over time, you cannot take a single snapshot of an event or intervention and say that it is the most common way something is done. Also, it does not mean that the leader of the organization knows what is right for the system today and again tomorrow. It does not mean that you can make useful, detailed, or long-range plans. It does not mean that you can promise specific outcomes within your organization within specific time frames. It does not mean that you can reach the level of professional competence and stop learning and growing. It does not mean that there is a set sequence of developmental stages that are predictable and controllable, and it does not mean that you can help the system transform without being transformed yourself.

What it does mean is that you need to participate as a self-organizing example. In the continuing emerging dynamics of a complex environment, you must be conscious of the conditions that affect the self-organizing processes and work with others to shape those conditions over time. You must be a learner and be responsible for complex self-organizing dynamics of yourself as a professional, and as you learn to engage with others, you must accept responsibility to help shape the conditions for emergent patterns for the larger picture, of which you are part.

Whole-system transformation

Transforming a system into a unified whole is the process of changing from one configuration into another by all parts and components of the system. For true transformation to take place, an organization must first function as a whole. If an organization has not achieved wholeness, it will separate into disconnected pieces and be unable to become whole again after the separation.

So what we mean by the term "whole-system transformation" is more than simply a change that affects the entire system. It literally means that the entire system is involved in creating itself all over again. This focus then moves from imposing change on the system from the outside to enabling or allowing the system to transform itself from the inside out. This type of transformation requires participants in the system to be self-aware of their environment and what is happening to them. They must understand their roles and what needs to be done when the transformation is complete. There needs to be an appreciation of all of the parts of the system and how they relate to each other and to the outside forces and environment that impact upon the system and that will either enhance or inhibit its change.

If these components are in place, the result is a healthy system that knows where to go next and can act quickly. Unfortunately, there are few "systems" that can do this. Many organizations are too "siloed" to effect any major system change. Any type of major transformation involves the organization as a whole, rather than working within very small segments of the organization. Whole-system transformation occurs only when there is a much larger and broader involvement and ownership of issues and responsibilities across the organization, rather than simply a focus on the executive suite or in smaller participating components of the organization.

Strategies for managing change

The discussion of managing transformation of the whole system can be overwhelming. But by breaking it down into its component parts, the series and processes can be adapted to any change that an organization, a unit, or smaller entity may want to make. Therefore, it is important that we understand some of the strategies for managing change throughout any particular change process.

As a leader, you need to decide now that every person involved in your change can and will play a critical role. Everyone within your organization plays a key role in interacting with each other. You can use some of the following strategies for organization or unit transformation:

Engage workers with their deepest-held values: Engage others as a group in the identification of what the most important values are to them. This can bind a group together for the pursuit of a common purpose. When there is a common purpose, the change process becomes a little bit more manageable and directable.

Articulate a bold vision and communicate it repeatedly: Communication through verbal conversations, e-mail, posters, memos, or other means is important in broadcasting the message. The organization's vision must inspire and bring forth the best of individuals in the organization. Keeping ourselves to a common vision increases the hope that the change will occur, and it nurtures people's creativity in assisting the process. Clarifying purposes of the change effort also helps to facilitate commitment and allows more people to participate on a grassroots level.

 A Practical Guide to Leadership Development

Invite others to participate in the realization of the vision: Establishing participative processes for strategic planning and supportive procedures for implementation and evaluation will help give people a common cause. Maintaining information flow, tapping resources, and meeting needs will also add to the change process. As we know, most learning is acquired by doing. Therefore, the participation of others provides an opportunity for using each other as a resource and results in the widest possible range of learning within the organization.

Be aware that there will be resistance: You must become comfortable and adept at managing resistance because participation enhances ownership. We know that even though we have invited multiple people to participate, resistance will always be present. The only thing that changes about resistance is its intensity and its manifestation. It must be addressed or it will become more extreme and your ability to make any changes will be seriously limited.

Do not hold individuals accountable for the entire system: Hold the entire system accountable instead. Everybody should be engaged as an experimenter and researcher in sharing new ideas in learning and problem solving.

Organizations of the future will be based on the principle of adaptability and their ability to change quickly rather than predictability. Organizations will be open; process will be more important than structure; and free human interaction will be more effective than impersonal chain of command hierarchies. As we move toward these types of organizations, it will be an intelligent, adaptable, learning organization that can respond rapidly to shifts in the changing social environment. It requires every individual who works in the organization to be receptive and willing to learn and help others to learn, and it requires every individual to accept responsibility for success in the organization. When we talk about large organizations, these may seem overwhelming. But as leaders and managers, it is our responsibility to work with others like us in our system to ensure that this occurs.

What possibilities are achievable if we work as a whole system? What do we gain by integrating divided parts of an organization? And why is it particularly important in these times to be able to achieve systemwide success? As organizations evolve, they tend to shift into more mechanical modes of thinking in response to their operating environment. We find this in older organizations or ones that have had a recent change of leadership from someone who has been in place for very long time. In many cases, a new leader will take over a unit or organization and not necessarily follow the structure that was in place before. What will happen in trying to choose a leader or successor is that most people involved in the selection process will choose someone who is more controlled and orderly and who will try to keep things the way they are. This may not necessarily be the right approach to choosing a new manager in an environment that is changing.

As you look toward the future of whole-system transformation, do not be afraid to challenge the status quo. Always ask yourself the question "What if?" By constantly challenging your mind and your ability to look outside of the box, you will find emerging areas of interest that will be dynamically important to you and your organization. Transformation is a dynamic journey, not an event, and it is characterized by key actions, important questions, critical decisions, and ways to evaluate progress at each step along the way. Remember the change process is never-ending.

If you review your quality assessment plan, your organization may use the PDCA methodology. As mentioned earlier, this approach emphasizes the continuing, never-ending nature of process improvement, and the cycle is a simple feedback loop. As you continue to use this methodology in creating substantive change, you will have an organization where continuous improvement is the norm and not the exception.

References

Blake, R. R., and J. S. Mouton. (1964). *The Managerial Grid.* Houston: Gulf.

Gardner, B. H., and Demello, S. (1993). "Systems thinking in action." *Healthcare Forum Journal* 36(4): 25–28.

Fiedler, F. E. (1967). *A Theory of Leadership Effectiveness.* New York: McGraw-Hill.

Maani, K. (2002). "Technology in healthcare: A summary of the NZIHM annual conference 2002—Technology: Adding value to health." *Health Care and Informatics Review* 6(4).

Pascal, R., Millemann, M., and Gioja, L. (2001). *Surfing the Edge of Chaos: The Laws of Nature and the New Laws of Business.* New York: Three Rivers Press.

Vroom, V. H. (2002). "Motivation and leadership decision making." *Thinkers,* March 2002.

Chapter 5

COMMUNICATION

Learning objectives

After reading this section, the participant should be able to:

- Identify common problems presented by written and verbal communication
- Determine strategies for improving communication

Written and verbal communication problems

The effectiveness of communication depends upon mutual trust between leaders and the people whom they lead. Both of these groups benefit from a humanistic approach when considering the potential effects on interpersonal relationships.

Communication and decision-making require follow-through to ensure understanding and implementation. When these processes are inadequate or ambiguous, behaviors become negative and block professional and departmental goal achievements. Staff activities become stagnant, and staff members become frustrated with the lack of direction or open communication. When these actions occur, staff will do only what they are told, which results in a lack of professional development, departmental creativity, cooperation, and personal development. When people are uncertain or lack information, every individual captures a wrong concept of the true situation. These types of stressful situations use an inordinate amount of energy that could be put to better use within the unit.

Understanding communication

To understand the ramifications of ineffective communication, it is important to understand communication in general. Communication is a circular and interactive process that involves the sharing of a question, information, an idea, or an opinion. Messages can be sent through written, verbal, and nonverbal means to somebody who receives the message. The receiver responds to the sender's message with his or her own perception of that message. Because of the uniqueness of everyone's personal values, attitudes, and cultural upbringing, what is received may not be the same as what is said. The potential for inaccuracy in communication is always present and breakdown can occur at any point.

The form of a message sent depends on the sender's intent to either share information or receive it. When we want to obtain information, we form questions. When giving directions for task completion, messages are stated, and often the best means for this is a written or electronic methodology.

Written messages are often more accurate than verbal because the sender puts more thought into composing the message. The precision in written messages is further enhanced by the practice of rereading before sending. In today's fast-paced e-mail environment, we all too often do not take the time to read through a message before we hit the Send button.

When composing an e-mail or other form of written communication, remember that the most accurate written messages always include answers to the five "w" questions: who, what, when, where, and why.

Verbal communication is much more common than written, but it has tremendous potential for inaccuracy because the receiver may not always hear what the sender is saying. Face-to-face communication is usually more accurate than communicating on the telephone or through another person, and the intended message may lose its impact and accuracy if a second or third party is involved.

LEADERSHIP TIP

Remember playing the game "telephone" when you were a child? How often was the answer accurate by the time it reached the last person on the line? It is always better to relay messages one-on-one so that the person receiving the message hears accurate information.

When communicating verbally, words should be chosen with care, giving attention to the vocabulary and level of comprehension of the receiver. The correct use of grammar also increases accuracy. With today's mobile communication devices, such as PDAs and cell phones, the use of correct grammar has frequently been cast aside in favor of speed. But care should be taken to ensure the message being sent will be received in the way that you intended. You also can use body language and tone intonations to help clarify your message. Nonverbal communication can emphasize the content of the message. This can be done by maintaining eye contact during transmission of the message, which allows you to observe the receiver for any behavior that indicates agreement, disagreement, or misinterpretation of what you are saying.

Following the transmission of the message, receivers interpret it and feed back information on what they think they heard. Interpretation of the message can also be influenced by the receiver's personal and professional attitudes and values, and the opinion of the person sending the message. We have all been in situations where we have watched a negative response to our message, and this includes head shaking, frowning, eye rolling, and looking away.

It is our responsibility to interpret feedback. The sender interprets the receiver's verbal and non-verbal responses. If the receiver's behavior indicates that the intended message has not been received or has been interpreted correctly, then the sender must go through the process again.

Formal and informal communication

There are two types of communication systems that exist in every organization: formal and informal. Formal communication is usually centered on a task or something that needs to be accomplished, whereas informal communication networks within organizations are usually socially connected. Informal communication is a primary way of establishing and maintaining interpersonal relationships both within and outside of work. An informal communication system is a network that can be established by individuals to exchange information or opinions, and it can be a very valuable tool to the manager as a source of information. There is an old adage that goes something like this: "Never cut down the grapevine!" Why? Because the grapevine is the informal communication network in many organizations, and it is where a majority of opinions, rumors, and misinformation can be obtained from the staff.

Although it is important to ensure you do not engage in the informal grapevine inappropriately—for example, by commenting on or indulging in gossip—it can be useful to keep one's ear to the ground. It's often the case that the staff members are the first to know about situations, before management really finds out about a formal problem or change. Informal communication systems are most active when formal communication systems do not operate with efficiency, speed, or accuracy, and this benefits neither staff nor management. Information on the grapevine is often inaccurate. When there are changes in policy, payday, personnel, or other major issues that affect an organization, the process puts pieces and parts together, in a fragmented and distorted way, and then passes them along to everybody else. Once again, the game of "telephone" has begun. These conversations usually begin with the words "Have you heard?" A good leader will remain in touch with the informal network so that correct information can be substituted for the inaccurate or distorted facts that will arrive from it. It is very important to keep staff members informed of any anticipated changes in an organization, to prevent the informal network from creating excessive tension or problems within the organization.

Ramifications of poor communication

Communication is a matter of perception, and it is by far one of the most important issues in any organization. Across all levels of any organization, it is difficult to ensure that everybody understands what is being said 100% of the time. From the lowest position up to the CEO, everyone assumes that they are understood because what they are saying is very clear to them. But too often what you say is not understood. When you begin to understand the way communication can be interpreted, it is easier to understand such things as why a police officer can get two opposing views of a crime scene from two different eyewitnesses, and how two people in an organization can have a fundamentally different view of a company's purpose, mission, and values, or how they can have a conversation and come away with totally different ideas about what has been said.

Assumption and feelings

So, it is important that we learn how to speak. If you want to become an effective communicator, you need to heighten your awareness of the human interaction that is involved in the communication process. In addition to perception, there are two other aspects of communication that you need to understand. The first is assumptions, and the other is feelings. Just as we assume that our messages are clearly received, we also assume that because something is important to us, it is important to someone else. That is why we assume that our leadership is accepted and everyone is looking at the problem the same way, or that our perception of reality is the only perception.

The problem with assumptions is that we never test them out. Over time, assumptions become facts because that is the way they land in our mind. Therefore, the first step toward good communication is to stop assuming that the other person understands exactly what you are trying to say just because you understand it.

Unfortunately, in some workplaces, it is generally accepted that there is no place for feelings. When dealing with the situations that we see every day in healthcare, we look for pure logic and think that communication has no feeling in it. On the contrary, people are dealing with our feelings all the time every day. If we are trying to communicate with somebody and do not think about the feelings involved, then we are missing half of the situation.

An easy way to find out about feelings is to ask the other person what they think and feel about a certain situation or the communication that you just gave them. The best way to handle feelings is to acknowledge them and then deal with them, instead of pretending that they are just not there. If we put someone on the defensive, which will happen if we do not deal with his or her total self, then communication will be blocked.

How do we prevent someone from blocking communication by defense? Here are some instances that cause the receiver to be defensive. Paying attention to these issues will allow you to correct and avoid them:

- The listener perceives the speaker's expression, tone of voice, manner of speech, or content to be critical

- The listener perceives the communicator as controlling

- Anything that is perceived by the listener to be manipulative, game playing, withholding information, or not playing it straight will also block communication

- The speaker shows no concern for the welfare of the other person

- The speaker has a poker face

- The speaker conveys an attitude of superiority

- The speaker is a know-it-all

Again, it is important to emphasize that not all the meaning in a conversation is in the words. If you are sensitive to the other person's movements or body actions, you will pick up important clues indicating that he or she may not have heard everything you said. However, it is very difficult to interpret exactly what every example of body language means. Never try to psychoanalyze someone based on his or her body language; instead, use it as a way to open up discussion to get at the right feelings and why the person is doing whatever he or she is doing.

Listening

Listening is the other side of talking when it comes to effective communication. Unfortunately, people rarely listen carefully to each other, and one reason for this is that receivers take in words much faster than speakers can speak them, so the receivers' minds begin to wander. They think about their response before they have heard the entire conversation, or they think about what they just did, what they have to do next, or whatever else pops into their minds. Essentially, receivers' minds wander and the next thing they know, they have missed two or three sentences, and half the conversation is gone.

Think about how often you have already formulated a response before the person finishes what he or she has to say. Often it is more than 50% of the time. But thinking of a reply and really listening to what is happening are mutually exclusive. Thinking about your response means you lose so much of what is being said, and you may miss subtleties and complexities because your mind has moved on. Sometimes we must force ourselves to listen to the entire conversation before we start thinking about our reply.

There are even more complex reasons for not listening. If you are really set in your view of the world, then truly listening to what somebody else has to say does not mean anything to you, because you are not going to change anyway. You might not listen because listening implies a willingness to accept another view.

 A Practical Guide to Leadership Development

Effective communication develops relationships

Communication is an interpersonal process, which means that becoming an effective communicator is not simply watching your language and cleaning up your delivery, it is also a matter of improving the manner in which you relate to people. One of the most important steps to becoming a good communicator is to develop an awareness of your own limitations and issues as a communicator. Do you tend to tune people out if they strike you the wrong way? How about if they are different from you? There are ways to address your communication limitations:

1. Be aware of your issues. Pay attention to how much or how little you hear of what people say.

2. Notice how often you make judgments about others in the early stages of communication.

3. Take careful notes of the problems brought to you, and think carefully about the nature of the problem.

This last point is a good tool to help you manage problems and develop your own communication skills. Keep track of the problems people bring to you. Are they technical issues, or ones that involve misunderstandings between individuals and groups? At the end of the day, evaluate how many questions came to you that were technical or clinical in nature and how many involved interpersonal relationship issues somewhere in your unit or the organization. As you move further in your awareness process, think about all your assumptions when you make a decision or give instructions that are going to affect other people.

Mean what you say and say what you mean

As a leader, it is very important to learn how to be direct without being abusive, condescending, or demeaning. Things left unsaid always lead to assumptions on the part of others, and we know that this blocks communication. Any time you have a communication void, it gets filled with an assumption based on somebody else's assumptions, not yours.

It is important when you speak to get it all out and get it all out honestly. People appreciate those who can give them straight talk. Communication must be honest, up-front, on the table, and direct. People may initially be surprised by this communication technique, because sometimes it is unusual to have everything on the table. But once they understand that this is where you are coming from, they acknowledge their relief at being able to communicate honestly and directly.

This honest and up-front communication must also be without retribution. Since people don't have to wonder where you are coming from, there is less fatigue and more energy put into their work and their play away from work. As you become more of an open and honest communicator, others in your ranks will too. The only way to deal with someone who is open and honest is to be open as well. It only takes one or two in any unit to start this communication style before the communication pattern will spread to others. An individual manager in one small unit can make a significant difference in an organization. Without open and honest communication, you will not be able to achieve anything else in your area.

What's the value in letting yourself out?

The ability to say how you feel, admit your fears and weaknesses, and acknowledge your mistakes is a sign of tremendous strength and a powerful communication device. People need to understand who you are, where you are coming from, and what you are made of.

In our society, and even in our educational upbringing, we are taught that to admit a mistake is to show weakness and to show any kind of a weakness is a bad trait, whether at a managerial or staff level. But managers need to be able to say that they don't know, or "Your idea sounds better than mine, so let's try it." Why? Because you will win the trust and support of your employees, and there will be a renewed trust in an environment where people can be who they are.

Show them your personal side

Most interpersonal relationships in organizations are position-to-position relationships, and it is rare that they are person-to-person relationships. In many organizations, managers speak in the role as the "boss" and they are treated as such; they have titles on their doors, desks, and business cards, all referring to their power position. The meaning behind this is "I want you to respect my position, regardless of who I am as a person."

The trouble with being a "position" rather than a person is that if you are talking to someone in your role, then you reform your statements, censor your feelings, and cover your tracks,

         A Practical Guide to Leadership Development

just to tell them what you think they need to know. But if you speak to someone as a person, then you trust your instincts, tell the other person how you feel, tell the whole story, and take responsibility for who you are, both as a person and as a leader.

Here are some small ideas that will help you be more personal:

✔ When interviewing someone, never sit behind a desk

✔ Ask people what they think, and tell them your concerns

✔ Never evaluate; always coach

✔ Be concerned for what someone can do for the organization, but also be concerned for him or her as a person

✔ Always be personal—your goal is to have people think of you as the person, not the position

Tips for written communication

How many times in your career have you opened up an e-mail or memo, read the contents, and become angry about them? How many times has an e-mail or memo put a damper on your happy day? If yours is like most organizations, the answer is often.

Today memos have mostly been replaced by e-mails, which have become the primary source of communication problems within the organization. Even e-mail is sometimes a one-way communication style, and this always runs a high risk of being misunderstood. Before writing an e-mail or putting anything to paper, always think carefully about the reaction that the missive will cause. Consider your own reason for writing it, and if you can call or tell the person face-to-face instead, it may be wise to do so.

Tips for active and sensitive listening

Are we really hearing what another person is saying? Are we sensitive to what our employees are saying? Are you encouraging and supporting? For new or improving managers, becoming effective listeners will go a long way toward encouraging and supporting your employees.

Listening well is one of the most effective ways to tell people that you respect them and that you care for them as individuals.

When we are listening to somebody, follow some of these simple rules:

✔ Never judge until you have all the facts.

✔ Expect that you will learn something when someone is speaking to you.

✔ Listen, not just to the words, but to the intended meaning of the statements. Look behind the words to see what they are actually saying.

✔ Always maintain eye contact with the person speaking.

✔ Use body language and facial expressions, such as nods and smiles, to assure speakers that you are in contact with them.

✔ Take responsibility for understanding the content and feelings of the communication. Respond in your own words to what you believe is a speaker's message. Always paraphrase the words that you understand, and hopefully the speaker will understand. This will give the speaker an opportunity to either acknowledge that you understand the meaning or clean up the statement so that you get the real message.

Tips for building successful work relationships

What does it take to make relationships work? The literature contains consistent themes that the evidence shows are crucial in building successful relationships:

- Trust
- Diversity
- Respect
- Effective communication

Trust: This is the foundation for every successful collaboration and relationship. People in trusting relationships seek input from each other and allow each other to do their jobs without interference and oversight. How do we gain trust? Open and honest communication is an excellent beginning.

Diversity: Diversity is essentially the differences in the way people view the world. It comes from differences in age, race, gender, education, experience, and thought. Diversity broadens the number of potential solutions, enabling people to learn from one another.

Respect: Respectful interactions are considerate, honest, and tactful. People who respect each other and value each other's opinions can willingly change their minds in response to what others say. Respect is especially important in very challenging situations, as it will help individuals focus on problem solving and communication.

Effective communication: Effective communication between individuals can be described as either rich or poor. Rich communication, such as face-to-face interaction or telephone conversations, is preferred for messages with potentially unclear meanings or with emotional content. Poor channels of communication, such as e-mails and memos, are preferred for more routine messages. In successful organizations, management and staff understand that both rich and poor communication channels are necessary and use each effectively.

Paying close attention to these factors can affect and influence the quality of work relationships and the environment, and leaders and managers can be much more effective in creating an environment where social and task-related relationships can thrive.

Be a champion of two-way communication. Be flexible and responsive by creating dialogue with the people who work for you and with you. It also helps to get frequent feedback from the people you deal with everyday about your communication skills. The key to improvement in patient care and any relationship is constant open and trustful communication. Making yourself available and giving your staff the shared control of communication processes will help you and your staff develop into better people and leaders, with the resulting effect of better-quality patient care.

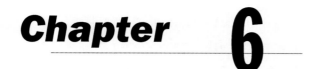

Chapter 6

BUILDING A POSITIVE
WORK ENVIRONMENT

Learning objectives

After reading this section, the participant should be able to:

- Examine factors in the healthcare workplace that hinder positive work environments
- Discuss strategies that create a healthy work environment
- Determine how organizational culture and climate affect leadership
- Describe how different leadership styles can be used to suit the situation

Fostering positive environments

Creating a positive environment for leadership development includes many areas of focus. This chapter focuses on establishing and sustaining healthy work environments and organizational climate and culture, engaging staff, fostering shared decision-making, and empowering and adapting your leadership style to the particular problem or environmental issue at hand.

It has been said that a positive work environment exists only when there is active interchange between an organization's leaders, managers, and employees. Occasionally leaders can achieve success independently of an organization that is not supportive of a healthy workplace. However, when the leaders and the organization are in sync, then many positive results and changes can be achieved. Today's healthcare workforce, with its myriad of shortages in skilled employees in every discipline, warrants an aggressive look at creating an environment where people will want to work and stay. Healthcare organizations that want to remain competitive need to retain a high-performing workforce.

Challenges of the healthcare workplace

The literature contains a great deal of discussion of the various challenges and workforce shortages. Jo Manion, in her book *Create a Positive Health Care Workplace! Practical Strategies to Retain Today's Workforce and Find Tomorrow's,* drew some conclusions about the challenges of workforce development and maintenance (2005):

1. **Workforce shortage:** Critical shortages of key workers in healthcare have occurred at various times, and shortages are likely to continue and possibly worsen in the future. In the recent past, shortages can be documented in several healthcare professional groups, including nurses, pharmacists, radiology technicians, physical therapists, and information technology managers. The impending retirement of baby boomers may significantly worsen the shortage, and it should be noted that the degree of shortages vary by geographic location and are occasionally cyclical in nature.

2. **Positive environment:** The creation of a positive environment is important regardless of whether there is a shortage of healthcare workers. The type of work environment directly affects the quality of customer service provided, the productivity of employees, and, eventually, the financial well-being of an organization. In most organizations, having a positive workplace increases the competitive edge.

3. **Reasons for shortage:** There are many well-documented reasons for the shortage. As we move forward through the new generations, there are fewer people available for recruitment, and many feel that healthcare is less attractive than other professions. As baby boomers age and become a greater percentage of healthcare users, the problem will become more complex and difficult to solve.

4. **Desire for good treatment:** Not every healthcare organization has a workforce shortage or experiences shortages in the same way. Sometimes healthcare

organizations note that the only difference between them and others like them is in the skills, knowledge, commitment, and abilities of the people who work for the organizations. Those organizations treat their employees well, but unfortunately there are just as many organizations that do not treat their employees very well and consider their replacement as simple as replacing equipment or supplies. There is a scarcity of talent out there, and many in the younger generations are unwilling to work for an organization that treats them poorly. Organizations that find themselves short on talent probably deserve to be that way.

Creating a culture of retention

If the marketplace for recruitment of healthcare professionals is going to be this difficult, then how do we create a climate that is not only healthy, but also allows us to retain and develop our employees in these difficult times? How does one "create a culture of retention"?

First, one must define this culture. A culture of retention can be considered an environment where people want to stay, where they enjoy work, and where they want to get involved. It is an organization where everybody works to make it a good place to work and where the environment meets people's needs. When employees come to work, they enjoy being there, feel good about it, feel safe, trust each other, and are confident that their jobs are done to the best of their ability.

How to create the culture

As a leader, how do you create this culture? In reviewing the literature, there are four areas that come into play. First, put employees first. Second, develop and cultivate authentic connections between you and your employees. Third, coach your employees toward higher levels of competence. Fourth, focus on getting results while partnering with employees. If leaders focus on these four areas, they can begin to create a culture of engagement.

1. **Put employees first:** Putting employees first allows them to focus on putting their patients first. How do managers put their employees first? The answer is simple: You should care about them, meet their needs, treat them with respect, express appreciation, listen, and provide support when they need it.

2. **Develop connections:** The second question is how to develop and cultivate authentic connections between you and your employees. Sharing some of yourself and letting them know that you care about them and the same things that they care about will invariably help to form a connection. By listening to them and getting to know them the same way they should get to know you, you will begin to develop a closer relationship. More importantly, you as a leader must create a sense of community, which you can develop over time, so that everyone working on your unit understands how important it is to be there and that they work to help each other.

Developing connections

Something that sounds quite simple, but that is vitally important, is hiring the right people—people who fit into your unit and your community. People's attitudes, behavior, and thinking skills will tell you whether they fit into the unit and the type of environment that you have created.

Another key to building relationships is to sometimes have fun. Fun can be had in a whole variety of ways. As a manager, I always try to keep it light-hearted and have a good sense of humor. In our business, it is difficult enough to provide the services we do, and so we should try to have fun doing it. I used to tell my staff that if they could not come to work and have fun, then they should just stay home, because the old adage that "one bad apple can spoil the whole bunch" is really true.

3. **Coach:** The third key is coaching and getting better competence from our staff. Setting high standards while supporting individual development is the most important thing that we can do to help our staff develop higher levels of competence. By modeling behavior and managing performance, as discussed in Chapter 7, we can begin to look for better results and engage employees in our units.

4. **Focus on results:** In any coaching situation, it is most important to focus on the results. When considering coaching, you do not necessarily need to worry about the process as much as you need to worry about the outcome. Always focus on the end game.

       A Practical Guide to Leadership Development

When attempting to create a culture of engagement, ask yourself these questions:

- ✔ What do you do to demonstrate that you put your employees first?
- ✔ How is the working relationship with your employees?
- ✔ Have you been able to make any progress in solving difficult problems?
- ✔ How much time do you spend working with your employees individually to help them move toward greater professional development?

Creating and sustaining healthy work environments

In 2005, the American Association of Critical-Care Nurses (AACN), in collaboration with some other organizations, joined together to complete the survey "Silence Kills: The Seven Crucial Conversations for Healthcare." Some of the key findings of the survey include (AACN 2005):

- Eighty-four percent of physicians and 62% of nurses and other clinical care providers saw coworkers take shortcuts that could be dangerous to patients.

- Eighty percent of physicians and 40% of nurses and other healthcare providers say they work with people who have shown poor clinical judgment.

- Fewer than 10% of physicians, nurses, and other clinical staff directly confront their colleagues about their concerns and issues, and one in five physicians say they have seen harm come to patients as a result.

- The 10% of healthcare workers who raise these crucial concerns observe better patient outcomes, work harder, and are more satisfied and committed to staying in their jobs.

Interestingly, about half of the respondents to the survey said that their concerns regarding these issues have lasted for a year and sometimes more. The study found that the prevalent culture of poor communication and collaboration among health professionals has contributed significantly to the continuance of medical errors and staff turnover. History shows that large gaps in communication and handoff can result in harm to patients. The report also says that better communication among healthcare workers who are confident in their abilities to raise their concerns results in higher satisfaction levels with their jobs.

The AACN has developed standards for establishing and sustaining healthy work environments. These standards provide a framework that promotes core competencies—such as communication and collaboration—ensure patient safety, enhance staff recruitment and retention, and maintain an organization's financial viability (AACN 2005).

The standards are as follows:

- **Skill communication:** Nurses must be as proficient in communication skills as they are in clinical skills

- **True collaboration:** Nurses must be relentless in pursuing and fostering collaboration

- **Effective decision-making:** Nurses must be valued and committed partners in making policy, directing and evaluating clinical care, and leading organizational operations

- **Appropriate staffing:** Staffing must ensure the effective match between patient needs and nurse competencies

- **Meaningful recognition:** Nurses must be recognized and must recognize others for the value each brings to the work of the organization

- **Authentic leadership:** Nurse leaders must fully embrace the imperative of a healthy work environment, authentically live it, and engage others in its achievement

Leaders who commit to these standards and work to implement them will be much more successful in retaining staff and creating the healthy work environments that are critical to patient safety and better patient outcomes.

Organizational climate and culture

In today's healthcare environment, organizational climate and culture play an important role in the success or failure of change initiatives and the creation of a healthy workplace. There has been much discussion about the difference between climate and culture, but in many ways they are really part of the same phenomenon, so this section will address both.

Organizational climate has been described as relatively temporary, subject to direct control, and limited to aspects of the organization that are consciously perceived by its membership—in other words, how it feels to work in a particular environment or what the atmosphere of the workplace is like. Culture, on the other hand, has been defined as an unconscious pattern of basic assumptions that a given group has identified and discovered, that were developed in learning to cope with the group's problems of external adaptation and internal integration, and that worked well enough to be considered valid, and therefore, to be taught to new members as the correct way to perceive, think, and feel as related to these problems (Schein 1991).

It is difficult to discuss climate and culture in anything but abstract terms. There have been significant studies looking at appropriate measures for climate and culture within organizations and on nursing units, but they have not found any particular style climate or culture that may be conducive to improving retention or creating a positive healthcare workplace. However, there appears to be consensus in the literature that organizational climate and culture may be two of the most important areas and that it is worth exploring the relationship between them and the nurse, patient, and organizational outcomes.

As a nursing leader, it is your responsibility to try and foster as positive a climate as possible in your particular area, even though the culture of your organization may not support that. The climate in individual areas can be good even if the overall culture around the organization is not supportive of the development of leadership and others within it.

Your leadership style matters

If empowering your employees is the key to treating them right and motivating them to treat your patients right, having a strategy to shift the emphasis from leader as boss to leader as partner is imperative. So, how do we know exactly what the right strategy or the right leadership style is at any particular time?

In the past, candidates for leadership positions were asked what type of leadership style they had, and there were only two answers: autocratic or democratic. This was a time when people believed that you were either one style or the other and could not be both, and there were numerous debates about the difference between democratic and autocratic leaders. Democratic managers and leaders were accused of being too soft, laid-back, and laissez-faire. Autocratic managers were often considered too tough, domineering, demanding, or even dictatorial to some degree.

Today, managers have a great deal more flexibility and are able to adapt leadership styles to situations. For example, if you have new employees on the unit, your leadership style will require you to provide a great deal of direction and focus on the tasks for the inexperienced employees. Conversely, those employees who are experienced and skilled require less hands-on supervision.

LEADERSHIP

TIP

If you look at all of your employees, you will find that they are all at different levels of development, depending on what you are asking them to do. You must evaluate them all separately.

Matching leadership style to people

To bring out the best in people and continue to create a healthy workplace environment, it is important to match the developmental level of the person being led with the required leadership style. Overall, giving too much or too little direction has a negative effect on an employee's development. This is why it is incredibly important to match leadership style to developmental level.

An effective strategy for managing this is Situational Leadership®, a leadership model originally created by Ken Blanchard and Paul Hersey at Ohio University in 1968. This particular model of leadership opens up communication and forces a partnership between leaders and the people who report to them. The model is based on the belief that people can and want to develop, and that there is no best leadership style to encourage the development. The model allows for tailoring the leadership style to the situation at hand.

Situational leadership includes four basic leadership styles (Blanchard, 1985):

 A Practical Guide to Leadership Development

1. Directing: corresponding to an enthusiastic beginner
2. Coaching: corresponding to a disillusioned learner
3. Supporting: corresponding to a capable performer
4. Delegating: corresponding to a self-reliant achiever

At this point, we can start thinking that leaders need to do what the people they supervise cannot do for themselves at the present moment. This is the premise of the entire model, and to become efficient and effective in using this model, you must master three skills: diagnosis, flexibility, and partnering for performance. None of the skills are difficult; each simply requires practice.

Diagnosis: The first skill, diagnosis, is something that healthcare professionals are very familiar with. In diagnosing the skills of one of your employees, there are two things to look for: competence and commitment. Competence is the sum of knowledge and skills that individuals bring to work. How well do employees report, plan, organize, problem-solve, and communicate about their work? Can they accomplish their goals and work on time? Competence is gained through formal education and experience, and is developed over time with appropriate direction and support. Commitment is people's motivation and confidence, and how interested or enthusiastic they are in doing their job. If they trust in their own abilities, motivation and confidence are high, and your direct reports are committed to the job.

Flexibility: As you develop the necessary skills for this particular model and reach a comfort level, then you have mastered the second skill of flexibility. Much like coaching, employees need to have different styles based on where they are in their own developmental model. Unfortunately, studies have shown that well over half of leaders tend to use only one style, one third tend to use only two styles, only 10% use three styles, and most importantly, only 1% use all four styles.

Partnering for performance: The third skill of the situational leader is partnering for performance. This skill opens up communication between you and your employees and increases the quality and quantity of conversations. When you begin to use the new model, make sure your employees understand how you are going to do it. They need to understand that you will be changing your style of management based on the developmental style of the people who work for you. Partnering involves give and take on the part of both leaders and followers. It is not something that you do *to* people, but something that you do *with* people.

Personal transformation

Developing effective leadership skills is a transformation. This type of leadership model applies not only to leading an individual, but also to leading teams, organizations, and, most importantly, yourself. The role you are in and your developmental level will change the style you need to use in each situation. Before you can lead anybody else, you need to know how to lead yourself and know what it takes to be successful. Introspection and knowledge of yourself will give you this perspective. Only leaders who have experience in leading themselves are ready to lead others.

One-to-one leadership

The key to one-to-one leadership is being able to develop a trusting relationship with others. If you do not know what your strengths and weaknesses are, you will not be able to develop a trusting relationship and will always keep the walls up, to keep you from being more vulnerable. Without some level of trust, it is impossible for any organization or person to function effectively. Trust between you and the people you lead is essential for a good working environment.

Team leadership

The next part of your development is team leadership, and most nurse managers are probably in this position now. As discussed earlier, preparation for team development and building a community of trust and empowerment are important parts of becoming an effective leader. It is important to honor the power of diversity and acknowledge the power of teamwork. This makes the leadership challenge more complicated, yet the results can be much more satisfying.

A big mistake made by leaders when they are promoted into a new position is to spend the majority of their time trying to improve things and change things at an organizational level before ensuring that they have faced their own credibility and their ability to manage a single team. If you think that major organizational change can occur without being comfortable with yourself or without having worked in a positive environment or created a positive environment, you are only fooling yourself.

LEADERSHIP

Don't try and fix everything at once. Start with something easy.

A Practical Guide to Leadership Development

While trying to develop new leaders or when in a new position as a leader yourself, it is important to create an environment that employees will enjoy working in. Do not make the mistake of trying to make too many changes at one time. It is best to spend some time looking at and listening to the organization before attempting to make any change at all. As a new leader, employees will come to you frequently with their individual agendas, and they will tell you what they think needs to be changed. One characteristic of an immature or new leader is to listen to everybody's complaints and then attempt to make all of the changes that have been requested. As a new leader in an organization, it is your duty to listen to what everyone has to say, make your assessment of what is happening on the unit, and then plan the change that you want to make. Communicate that change, and tell people why that change will improve the environment in which they work.

Identify issues you see in your newly assigned area. The earlier you begin to identify issues that you see, the more objective they are. At this point, you are still an outside observer to that particular organization or role. After a few months in the role, you will not be as objective and things will not look as new as they looked in the beginning. Take the time to write down everything that you see. After you write down what you see, you can make an action plan to begin to understand what's happening in the unit.

LEADERSHIP TIP

Looking, listening, and feeling the pulse of the area will give you the direction that you need to create an environment that is empowering, engaging, and fun to be at on a daily basis.

Simple rules to follow

Following these simple rules will help you succeed in creating a positive environment and becoming a better leader:

- ✔ Know yourself.
- ✔ Manage yourself.
- ✔ Trust yourself.
- ✔ Don't stand on ceremony.
- ✔ Don't be too impressed with yourself.
- ✔ Yes, you can be replaced.
- ✔ Take a time out if you need to; give time outs to people who look like they need it.
- ✔ Be comfortable with who you are, and always be the same person.
- ✔ Laugh at yourself.

✔ Make mistakes and then acknowledge that that's what they were.

✔ Remember, you were one of them once.

✔ Treat your employees like you want to be treated.

✔ Let other people make decisions.

✔ Ask for advice and then follow it. Don't ask for it if you don't intend to follow it.

✔ Be real; being someone you're not is transparent.

✔ Learn something new every day and then tell your employees what you learned.

✔ Ask your employees, "How am I doing?"

By following some of these rules, you will quickly learn who you are and so will your employees. Once you have crossed the line into leadership, you will be amazed at how the relationships between you and your employees change. It is important that you always be your real self. Never try to be somebody at work who is different from somebody outside of work. If you are not real, your employees will see right through you. Everyone has inherent skills built into themselves that they can transfer between home, work, and other environments in which they interact. If you are comfortable with who you are, what you know, and what you do, then it's very simple to be the same person all the time. It's also a lot easier!

References

American Association of Critical Care Nurses. (2005). "New study finds U.S. hospitals must improve workplace communication to reduce medical errors, enhance quality of care." Aliso Viejo, CA: Author.

American Association of Critical Care Nurses. (2005). "Communication in the healthcare workplace: A prescription for better care. Frequently asked questions." Aliso Viejo, CA: Author.

Blanchard, K. (1985). *Leadership and the One-Minute Manager.* New York: William Morrow and Co.

Manion, J. (2005). *Create a Positive Health Care Workplace! Practical Strategies to Retain Today's Workforce and Find Tomorrow's.* Chicago: Health Forum, Inc.

Schein E. H. (1991). "What is culture?" In P. J. Frost, L. F. Moore, M. R. Louis, C. C. Lundberg, and J. Martin (Eds.), *Reframing Organizational Culture.* Newbury Park, CA: Sage.

Chapter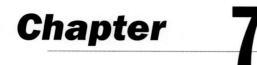

PROFESSIONAL DEVELOPMENT

Learning objectives

After reading this section, the participant should be able to:

- Explain the concept of performance management
- Discuss how leaders can use the concept of performance management to aid the professional development of staff
- Identify ways to resolve performance problems
- Discuss the use of coaching to improve employee performance and development
- Explain how mentors can influence employees' professional development

Components of professional development

Three of the most important tools you can use to encourage the professional development of your staff and help them become good managers and leaders are mentoring, coaching, and performance management. By using performance management to improve productivity, motivation, and morale, you will create a work environment that helps employees succeed.

Performance management

Performance management is concerned with having everybody succeed and improve. To make this happen, managers and employees have to work together in an open communication process that identifies barriers to success. Barriers can result from employees or the work system, so performance management involves planning to overcome these barriers.

Annual program ratings and yearly reviews lack the level of detail necessary to make this happen, unless managers are very competent and experienced in what they do to make the performance management program successful. Managers should focus 90% of their individual personnel improvement plan on continuous performance planning and communication throughout the year.

Communicating with employees

The development of specific and measurable objectives for employees is one of the most important steps in achieving success. It is the goal of managers to find ways to make performance better, and sometimes that means managers and employees need to figure out the best method to use for their individual situations on the unit. In planning performance development meetings, managers should ask employees what things have made their job more difficult and what they need to collectively do over the next year to help employees become more productive.

Many times we focus our performance management discussions on the past deficits of employees and areas that need to be improved. Instead, this discussion should take the other direction and be forward-thinking. Discussion should revolve around workflow, communication, and teamwork within the unit.

Managers should take the time to hold informal, short discussions with employees every month or so. These meetings can last for just a few minutes, but should focus on talking to employees about how things are going. Quarterly discussions can be more organized, and a year-end review should be just that, a review. However, remember that by the time of the yearly review, every issue should have been discussed previously, with no surprises.

Holding informal discussions lasting five to 10 minutes every month with employees helps you stay connected and in touch.

Establishing a communication system to get top performance and value from each employee requires individual attention to those employees. There is no one right plan for everyone.

When talking about performance with employees, it is important to be forward-looking, to place no blame, and to problem-solve. Continue to hold ongoing communication with employees and allow no surprises. The forms that managers fill out at the end of the year tend to lack relevance to the real purpose of performance management. When discussing performance, whether good or bad, we need to consider all barriers to employees' success.

Establish expectations

Performance management begins when jobs are initially defined, and it ends when an employee leaves the company. Between those two points, a working performance management system should include the following items:

- Clearly developed job descriptions
- An appropriate selection process
- Clear expectations
- Appropriate education, training, and orientation
- Consistent feedback and coaching
- Frequent performance development discussions
- Appropriate compensation and recognition systems
- Career development opportunities
- Knowledge of why employees leave the organization
- Encouragement of potential managers and supervisors

Clearly developed job descriptions: This is the first step in selecting the right person for the job and setting that person up to succeed. Job descriptions should provide a framework so that applicants and new employees understand the expectations of the position. Objectives should be expressed as outcomes. What do we actually expect to see in the performance of an employee?

An appropriate selection process: It is important to have an appropriate selection process. People have different skills and interests, and jobs have different requirements. Selection is the process of matching skills to the requirements of the job. Finding the best fit for someone is exceptionally important, and using a selection process that maximizes input from both management and potential coworkers may be the best thing that managers can do for their unit and their coworkers.

Clear expectations: Be sure new hires know exactly what they're supposed to do. One of the first reasons why people fail to meet your expectations and outcomes is because they do not know exactly what they are supposed to do. Therefore, developing clear job descriptions with outcomes, as mentioned earlier, is the most important piece of getting the right person in the right job.

Appropriate education, training, and orientation: You must provide appropriate education, training, and orientation. Before an employee can do a job, he or she needs to understand how to do it and have the necessary information in order to perform effectively. This would include any information and training that is job related, or company-related information that will help individuals perform better within the total organization. An understanding of the process, politics, and purpose of an organization and complete knowledge about the customer needs and requirements will lead to better retention and success of employees when they begin employment.

Consistent feedback and coaching: Providing consistent feedback and coaching is vital, as everyone needs ongoing and consistent feedback that addresses both strengths and weaknesses. Effective feedback focuses intensely on helping build on employees' strengths and not on criticizing their weaknesses. However, remember that feedback is a two-way process. Create a work environment in which people feel comfortable asking the question "How am I doing?" and create an environment where people are not afraid to hear how they are doing. This ensures that employees hear feedback that comes in both positive and negative formats.

Frequent performance development discussions: Conduct frequent performance development discussions and meetings with employees. When supervisors give employees frequent feedback and coaching, this can affect performance reviews. Providing supportive information regarding the positive performance of employees, and providing it frequently, lets employees know how they are performing in meeting their next goals and challenges. As we try to develop new leaders and managers within our staff, frequent performance development discussions and meetings become even more important. If people do not know where they stand, where they may have issues that need improvement, or how to enhance the positive skills that they do have, their advancement to managerial and leadership positions will be ever more difficult.

Appropriate compensation and recognition: Provide appropriate compensation and recognition systems. Although this may be outside of your control, it is important that the organization you work for provides an efficient and motivation-related payment system. If there is a system for rewarding merit shown through excellent performance, a fair and objective evaluation system must be in place in order to award those dollars.

Career development opportunities: Provide promotional and career development opportunities for staff. Managers and leaders play a key role in helping their staff develop their potential for growth into positions like yours. Growth, goal setting, challenging job assignments, responsibility, and cross-training all help the development of more efficient and effective staff members. The exposure to other departments and operations within the organization will help create an environment in which people feel more comfortable to experiment and make mistakes. The more employees see of the organization and understand its operation, the more valuable they will be to that organization.

Knowledge of why employees leave the organization: When skilled and valuable employees leave your organization, it is necessary to understand why. The feedback from these people will help you and your organization improve its work environment for those valuable people. An improving work environment results in retention of valued staff. If you truly create an environment that encourages discussion and feedback, and you meet regularly with your staff, you should learn nothing new in an exit interview.

Encouragement of potential managers and supervisors: Encourage potential managers and supervisors to take responsibility for managing performance and their work area, and promote cooperation for performance improvement across an organization. Help them understand that success in your work area, shift, or department contributes to the overall healthiness of the organization and creates a place where people want to work.

Handling performance problems and employees

Employees do not always do what you want them to do. Sometimes they act as competent professionals and other times they procrastinate, miss deadlines, and wait for instructions. Sometimes they blame others when their work is not up to par. Occasionally employees become defensive when you try to coach them to perform goal-meeting work.

If this scenario fits your unit, then performance management is the answer to your problem.

Reasons for poor performance

Open communication can help you find out exactly why employees are not meeting expectations. It is the responsibility of managers and leaders to identify what is wrong with the employees' function and how to correct it. The easiest issues to solve revolve around the tools employees need to do their job, the time to do it correctly, and the training and education to effectively manage what they do. If you do not provide these three things, employees will move on to an organization that will.

When trying to diagnose performance problems, consider the following items. Reviewing these simple questions will help you zero in on the problems that are causing poor performance:

- What issues regarding the present work system may be causing this person to fail?

- Have you discussed with the employee exactly what you want him or her to do? Do employees know the goals and the outcomes that are expected within their position? Do they share the same vision with you for the end result?

- Is the employee confident in his or her ability to perform the job? Procrastination usually results from the employee lacking confidence in his or her ability to produce an outcome, or it can result from the employee being overwhelmed with the magnitude of the task and not having the tools to perform it. This particular issue is common with new graduates or people who are moving to a new clinical area with which they are unfamiliar.

- Does your staff have the appropriate and necessary people working with them to accomplish their goals? Are these other members of the team keeping their commitments? If they're not, is there something that you can do to help them? For

 A Practical Guide to Leadership Development

example, are the ancillary departments—such as pharmacy, dietary, and housekeeping—supporting the clinical delivery of services within your area? You have a responsibility as a leader or a manager to intervene to change that process.

- Does your staff understand how their work fits into the larger picture of the organization? Do they appreciate the value of what they do? Sometimes staff members do not understand their role in the big picture of the organization and how important their work with individual patients on the unit is to the success of the organization. Such things as decreased length of stay, quick and efficient movement of patients through the system, no delays in testing or procedures, and other things that affect the efficiency of the organization turn out to be the responsibility of the individual staff on those units.

- Does your staff know what constitutes success? Perhaps they think that what they are contributing is good work and that you are an overly micromanaging supervisor. Or do they know what they are contributing to the organization? Do they feel valued and recognized for the work that they contribute? And do they feel fairly compensated, rewarded, and recognized for their contribution to the organization?

By reviewing these issues, an enabling manager will help employees succeed. By following these steps, answering the questions truthfully and honestly, and reviewing them with yourself and employees, you can help employees succeed and retain them in your organization. By establishing a baseline of performance management, you have adopted one of the best tools for encouraging and coaching your employees' success at work.

Strategies for resolving poor behavior

How do we handle problem behavior among our employees? Some of the most problematic behaviors we will see are absenteeism and tardiness, insubordination and uncooperativeness, and alcohol and drug abuse. We will discuss two general methods to help supervisors improve employee performance: counseling and a discipline process.

LEADERSHIP

TIP

Counseling can help employees solve their own problems. Discipline corrects or prevents unsatisfactory behavior.

Counseling helps employees solve their problems, which enables them to perform better at work. Supervisors should counsel employees when they need help in determining how to re-solve a problem that is affecting their work. When employees have problems that supervisors are unqualified to help with, they should refer employees to a professional.

Supervisors should administer discipline promptly, privately, impartially, and unemotionally. All disciplinary action should be documented and placed in an employee's file. Positive discipline focuses on preventing behaviors from ever beginning. This includes making sure employees know and understand the rules, creating conditions under which employees are least likely to have problems, and rewarding desirable behavior. The goal of positive discipline is really self-discipline among employees who voluntarily follow the rules and meet performance standards. Supervisors who expect self-discipline from their employees must practice it themselves. To best help their employees, supervisors should learn about their organization's procedures and resources for assisting employees. This may involve referring employees for help outside the organization or to the organization's employee assistance program should the behaviors be related to a possible substance abuse problem.

LEADERSHIP

TIP

Any time you have cause to discipline an employee, be sure to document the action in the employee's personnel record.

Common types of problem behaviors

In general, problem employees fall into two categories. First, there are employees who cause problems by starting fights, leaving early, or coming in late. Second, there are employees whose money worries cause distraction from work or who have such overwhelming problems at home that they cannot cope. By handling such employees appropriately, supervisors can help resolve the problem without hurting the morale or the performance of other employees. When supervisors observe poor performance, they tend to blame the employee for lack of ability or effort. But when explaining their own poor performance, both supervisors and em-ployees tend to blame the organization or another person for not providing enough support.

To uncover the true source of a performance problem, a supervisor might consider the following issues:

- Has this employee performed better in the past?

- Has the employee received proper training?

- Does the employee know and understand the objectives he or she must accomplish?

- Is the supervisor providing enough support and feedback?

- Has the supervisor encouraged and rewarded high performance?

- Are other employees with similar abilities performing well or experiencing similar difficulties?

Absenteeism or tardiness

Absenteeism and tardiness are expensive problems. The employee may be paid for the time off or replaced with a less productive person. Missing work is often a sign of a deeper problem, such as a family crisis, anger about something at work, or future plans to leave an organization.

Insubordination and lack of cooperation

Insubordination and uncooperativeness are two issues that not only affect the individual but also the entire work environment. Insubordination, which is a deliberate refusal to do what a supervisor or other superior asks, may result from not understanding how to do something. This can be corrected by training. Sometimes an employee performs poorly or breaks rules because he or she chooses to do so. This may be uncooperative behavior or a deliberate refusal to do what he or she is supposed to do.

Many kinds of negative behavior fall into the following categories:

- General poor attitude, criticizing, complaining, and showing dislike for the supervisor and organization.

- Making an art out of doing as little as possible by spending most of the day socializing, joking around, or moving as slowly as possible.

- Regularly failing to follow rules. This may be forgetting to wear safety equipment or sign in or out on time or just generally doing something that he or she knows is against the rules of the organization.

- Disregarding the supervisor's instruction to do something, saying that it will be done later. Sarcastic, hostile, or passive behavior may be a symptom of an underlying problem.

Alcohol or drug abuse

Alcohol or drug abuse may result in poor performance, such as unsafe practices, sloppy work, or frequent absences. These employees are expensive and dangerous to an organization. They can hurt the organization by lowering productivity, raising the number of unfortunate patient incidents, or even stealing services and/or supplies. These employees are more likely to quit, cause accidents, have a higher use of disability and sick time benefits, and increase insurance costs. Managers and leaders should note that the federal antidiscrimination law treats substance abuse as a disability and companies are encouraged to direct employees to get help. Any action taken with regard to employees should focus on work performance, not on the substance abuse itself. Since leaders and managers are responsible for ensuring a safe workplace for employees and others, if an employee suspected of substance abuse is creating a hazard, the manager must act.

Poor performance related to drinking may be more difficult for a manager to confront than illicit drug use. Drinking is socially acceptable; problem drinking behavior generally is not well understood; and the manager may sympathize with the employee who has a drinking problem. For example, a manager may overlook poor performance when he or she knows the employee is suffering from a hangover. To counteract this tendency, managers must be aware and take action. Additionally, managers should be aware of signs of drinking and drug use that can impair performance.

Theft

Employee theft includes the taking of company supplies, inventory, and other resources, such as time. Managers must take measures to prevent and react to theft. In addition to organizational procedures, managers should carefully check the background of anybody they plan to hire. They should make sure that employees follow all procedures for recordkeeping. They should also build employee morale and involvement, making sure employees understand the

         A Practical Guide to Leadership Development

costs and consequences of theft, and they should set good examples. When managers suspect an employee of stealing, they should report it to their superiors.

Counseling for poor performance and behaviors

If managers respond to a problem behavior immediately, they will sometimes be able to bring the problem to a quick end without complex proceedings. Often the most constructive ways managers can address the problem behavior is through counseling, or through learning about an individual's personal problem and helping him or her resolve it. For simple problems such as tardiness resulting from keeping late hours, calling the problem to the employee's attention may lead to a solution without additional help. For more complex problems, such as financial issues, personal relationship issues, or substance abuse, the employee should get expert help. In either case, counseling is a cooperative process between the supervisor and employee.

When counseling employees, start the interview with a discussion of the problem. Counseling often takes place as a result of employees' personal problems, and so they may be emotional during counseling sessions—be prepared for emotional or angry outbursts. Managers and leaders should remain calm and reassure employees that emotions are not innately good or bad.

The next step in the interview is to consider possible solutions. Rather than simply prescribing a solution, managers can usually be more helpful by asking employees questions that will help them come up with ideas and solutions of their own. When both agree on a solution, the manager should restate it to make sure employees understand.

Schedule a follow-up meeting after just enough time has passed for employees to begin seeing some results. At this meeting, managers should review their plans and discuss whether the problem has been, or is being, resolved. If this does not result in any change in employee performance, a disciplinary process may have to be put into place.

Disciplinary processes are usually specific to an organization, and your individual procedures for the disciplinary process should be followed. When managers have problems with the performance and behavior of employees, it is paramount that they take immediate corrective action to ensure that problems do not affect the entire unit or area where the employees work. Do not allow one person with a problem to infect the entire organization.

How do we help correct some of these issues before they become serious problems? One methodology is through coaching and goal setting. Coaching for improved performance will help avoid the disciplinary process and actions.

Coaching to improve performance

Problems should be regarded as opportunities to do better and gain experience. We learn best not by being taught or by studying or reading, but by experiencing, experimenting, and then reflecting on what we did, what happened, and drawing conclusions. If we don't learn from the past, we are doomed to repeat the same mistakes and have the same problems that we've always had. If this happens, we never grow and develop as a person and will effectively stagnate both emotionally and intellectually.

A technique for coaching someone is known as "commend, recommend, commend." Let's look at a sample of how this works. First, commend employees on any significant work duties that have been carried out well. This will help set the tone of the meeting and defuse any hostility. Be careful not to sound too patronizing. This first part is the commendation.

Now the recommendation part:

✔ Get straight to the point.

✔ State why you're having a conversation.

✔ Describe any behavior that is causing the problem.

✔ Explain the consequences of the behavior.

✔ Tell how the behavior makes you feel as a manager.

✔ Ask for employees' views. Ask them to assess their own behavior.

✔ Review employees' job competency requirements. As an example, check their understanding of their job description to ensure that you both have the same expectations.

✔ Ask employees how they will correct the behavior and how they can convince you that they will do it.

✔ Ask employees to say in their own words what specifically they will do to change their behavior. What outcome can you anticipate if this employee is successful in making the changes?

✔ Decide on the actions that the employee will take. Summarize your agreements.

Finish the meeting with another commendation and a positive comment. It is vital to end any conversation on a positive note, because the last thing that you say to anyone is what will be remembered the longest. You must respect employees' dignity and not undermine their self-confidence, which would reduce their commitment to change and create hostility and general apathy in the work environment. If employees feel valued, they will want to change; if they feel undervalued, they will not care.

We can use the coaching methodology in a variety of situations, such as for development of interpersonal or self-management skills or other clinical skills necessary in the unit. If there is a performance problem with problematic behavior and new challenges, we can also use the coaching situation. Finally, we can use the coaching situation for career development and to give people competencies they need for the future. Coaching is appropriate when there is a need to deal with a steep learning curve.

Benefits of coaching

How can you help someone as a coach? Coaching can help focus attention, create self-discipline, validate data, help share new ideas, and support the learning process. Conversely, you should not use the coaching situation when employees should leave an organization, such as when they are in the absolute wrong job. If people have significant personal problems, it is not appropriate to use coaching methodology.

In addition to the "commend, recommend, commend" style, there are also several steps to the coaching process. These steps are:

1. **Contracting:** What does the person want the coach to do and what are the expectations of both parties? Establish boundaries.

2. **Initial goal setting:** Goals should be made and clarified regarding what (knowledge), how (skills), and why (value). Standards should be set high.

3. **Assessment:** Observe and analyze current performance.

4. **Implementation:** Practice is the key to mastery. Implement the plan and continuously follow up.

5. **Action planning:** Give feedback on practice and performance.

6. **Final evaluation:** Follow up, summarize, and evaluate if goals have been achieved.

Overall, coaching is an excellent way to improve performance of your staff and help develop new leaders. It pays to coach rather than discipline your staff, but it is important to coach them in a way that makes them aware of the consequences of their own actions. Allowing them to tell you what they will do to change behaviors is important in keeping the communication process open. By applying this methodology, you are empowering your employees with the responsibility of changing their own behaviors, and that makes them feel directly accountable and involved in the situation, problems, and outcomes. A feeling of being involved makes employees feel committed to any changes required and, almost without fail, will result in higher levels of motivation and improved performance in your organization.

Adapting this style in today's healthcare environment is not an easy task. It takes work and time, but by taking some of these tasks into the coaching arena, you will become more and more successful in improving performance without discipline.

Mentoring

In nursing, mentoring is viewed as a professional obligation, a necessity of the work environment, and a way to attract and retain talent. The best organizations are those that grow their own people and grow their own leaders. A mentoring leader creates an environment that encourages the development of both individual and group mentoring relationships.

 A Practical Guide to Leadership Development

Mentoring relationships are particularly important during the development of new managers and leaders, as well as during transition points in someone's career. When you decide that one of your staff is going to be manager, it is critical that you ensure the person has a mentor to guide and support him or her through the process.

There are many articles and research studies that support the benefits of mentoring relationships during the periods of time when staff are preparing for leadership roles, a change in career or position, and at times when personal and professional satisfaction is needed.

Developing mentoring relationships

Mentor relationships can happen in both informal and formal settings. Informal mentor relationships occur through shared interests and goals, a mutual desire for something to happen, and the chemistry that may occur between the two people. The mentoring connection is a developmental and empowering relationship that extends over a period of time. During this time, learning and growth occur in a respectful and collegial atmosphere.

More formal mentoring relationships look a lot like coaching relationships. Generally, mentoring functions as a cyclical relationship, in which people enter the beginning of the cycle as mentees and leave the cycle as mentors.

Mentoring relationships progress along several steps:

1. Choosing a mentor
2. Becoming acquainted
3. Setting goals
4. Growing the relationship
5. Evaluating success

1. **Choosing a mentor:** The first step is choosing a mentor. The people who work for you may not necessarily choose you as their mentor and you may not choose them as mentees. It is important that the relationship be developed carefully and with great thought, because mentoring requires commitment and time as well as a relationship that is open and respectful.

2. **Becoming acquainted:** The next step is the getting acquainted component. Both parties need to define their expectations up-front and decide how communication in meetings will occur. Sometimes formal mentorships last for years; others last for shorter periods of time. It is at this point that the mentors and the mentees must agree on the relationship and the expected outcomes. In some cases a contract can be drawn up. It is also important at this point to understand that confidentiality is important in the relationship.

3. **Setting goals:** The third step is to set goals for the outcomes of the relationship. The major theme at this point will be "What do I want to get out of this?" At this point, mentees may want to assess their skills and then decide, with the mentor, what skills they need to learn. Whatever those skills are, they should be put in writing to ensure that the mentors and mentees are in agreement.

4. **Growing the relationship:** The fourth stage is growing a relationship. This is the longest phase of the relationship, during which both mentor and mentee meet regularly to review goals and adjust them as necessary. It is also the time when the problems within a relationship must be discussed. Should there be a situation where problems cannot be resolved, the best option may be to end the relationship.

5. **Evaluating success:** The last step is ending the relationship and evaluating its success. Most formal relationships come to an end when mentees have accomplished all of their goals, or they have been promoted or changed into the job for which they were being mentored. The end of the relationship requires some form of celebration. Mentors and mentees should also evaluate the relationship's success. Were the goals met? Was the outcome successful? What worked and what didn't? All of the answers to these questions should be committed to writing so that both parties will retain the lessons learned when they move into other relationships. We all learn by our mistakes, and we should remember what they were so that we can improve our relationships as we move forward.

When mentoring goes bad

Mentoring is not always successful. It is intended to help guide the development of an employee, but not all mentoring results in the growth of mentees. Mentoring can sometimes be a method of continuing past practices because it obstructs necessary changes to the work environment.

Some mentees believe that they should not seek out a wiser, older, experienced leader as a guide to what happens in an organization, but rather that a new leader should read a lot, listen, work, and observe. In this way, young leaders learn a lot on their own and are not given the antiquated wisdom gained from someone else's past. It has been said that "the workplaces of America are filled with industrious and upright citizens on a treadmill to nowhere, because they are so intent on playing it safe" (Porter-O'Grady and Malloch 2007).

Toxic mentoring can also result when aspiring leaders seek to please someone whom they have known for a long time or who is already experienced. If experienced leaders do not assist aspiring leaders in developing their own identities and styles, then aspiring leaders could be misled into following the same path as established leaders. Once the established leader is no longer on hand, a new leader might become empty and powerless and unable to progress because of the assimilation of the older leader's style.

It is also important not to place unrealistic hopes on anyone that you mentor. A good mentor will tell aspiring leaders that they must take initiative rather than try to travel the same old routes. It is important for mentees to expose themselves to positive environments, learn from the failures of their predecessors, and to seize opportunities rather than retreat from them when the pressure is on.

Leaders and mentors should take care not to simply select people and promote those who are a reflection of their own image. It is important that experienced leaders choose individuals who exhibit strong qualities, represent a diversity of personalities, and demonstrate critical-thinking skills that will enable them to create solutions to the significant problems that may arise in their institutions.

References

Livingston, J. S. (1988). "Pygmalion in management." *Harvard Business Review* 66(5), 121–130.

Porter-O'Grady, T., and Malloch, K. (2007). *Quantum Leadership: A Resource for Healthcare Innovation*, 2nd edition. Boston: Jones and Bartlett Publishers.

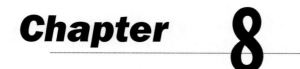

Chapter 8

CHANGE MANAGEMENT AND PROJECT LEADERSHIP

Learning objectives

After reading this section, the participant should be able to:

- Explain the concept of change management
- Examine the role leaders can play as change agents
- Discuss ways to create an environment that supports change
- Explain the role of a project manager
- Determine strategies that will help projects become successful

Change management

Change means to alter, become different, or to transform. Changes occur in organizations as a result of forces that affect the organization, both internally and externally, and these forces can act on individuals or the organization as a whole.

External forces are those forces that originate outside the person or the organization, and include such things as changes from government, insurance companies, consumers, or competitors. Internal forces are those forces that work within an organization, and may include new policies and procedures, movement of units, or other issues that affect what we do as managers and leaders.

Leaders' roles as change agents

As managers and leaders in healthcare organizations, it is our responsibility to be change agents. A change agent is a person who causes or creates change, and this person may originate the change or may be one who recognizes the value of new ideas that are generated by others. Managers who are able to embrace and lead change, rather than resist it, will be positioned for an interesting and successful career.

If you are a change agent or are responsible for leading a change, you may be called a "champion of the cause." Others affected by the change can be referred to as "stakeholders." As a champion, it is the manager's responsibility to enable change. Change is a reality that we must accept and, as the manager, it is our responsibility to enable it and help it occur.

Before any change can occur, the manager should assess the situation and the considered change. There are many things to consider:

- Assess the difficulties or problems that the change is designed to alter
- Assess where the changes are coming from
- Assess who supports the potential for change and who is critical of it
- Assess who will gain from the change and who will lose

LEADERSHIP

TIP

If you expect the change to be resisted, it is critical that you understand why.

Resistance can be found in multiple points, from the presentation to the timing or pace of the change. Occasionally, there may be resistance because the proposed change is weak. In some cases, groups affected by the change may be unwilling to give up benefits or things such as policy and procedure that they have had in the past.

Resistance to change

Resistance to change is probably the major roadblock when trying to transform any organization. Inertia, habit, and comfort all contribute to resistance to change. Most people prefer established routines and therefore do not actively seek out change. Routine provides us with control, and because change is sometimes ambiguous and the outcomes are not always known, it takes away control.

People involved in change want to know why, when, and how the changes will occur, and they also want to know how it's going to affect them. Managers have to take extra effort to accomplish change so that it is adequately explained to those involved; otherwise, the change has little chance of success. By explaining the outcome of the change, you will gain the trust of the people involved and decrease the resistance that you may encounter.

Reasons why change is resisted

The following are reasons why change may be resisted:

- Poor timing
- Poor presentation of the proposal
- Weak proposal
- Poor timing and pace of the change process
- Lack of trust
- Loss of control
- Taking people out of their comfort zone

So how do we know when change is being resisted? The most obvious way is active and vocal opposition to what is happening. Less obvious, and more dangerous, is passive resistance, where people resist by not doing what needs to be done and continuing with the old processes and policies. Some people may be indifferent to the change, and others may try to make the change but never get it quite right.

Plan for change

Before attempting to make any change, have a plan in place. Groups that experience success in one change are usually willing and able to take on other changes. As a manager,

---

it is important to empower the people who work for you with the ability to make an effective change. Having a positive attitude, empowering your staff, communicating well, and describing the plan and its perceived outcomes will help you be successful.

There are several factors to be addressed when planning a change:

- Time the change appropriately.

- Consider the speed of change.

- Consider the scope of the project.

- Develop trust with those involved in the change by communicating all components and parts of the plan and encouraging full participation.

- Make sure to listen to those involved.

- Encourage the involvement of all staff. Having them involved will give them a sense of control in developing the new process.

- Demonstrate your own commitment to the change. When your staff sees that you are part of the change and encouraging it, they will be more committed to work with you to make it happen.

- Provide appropriate resources and support. Any change that is underfunded, undervalued, or given too little time to work will be a failure.

Even after using these techniques to get everyone on board, you will still find people who are resistant to the change, so you may need to enlist a few other approaches and techniques to get staff to buy into your plans.

The first of these approaches is negotiation. If you are dealing with a unionized environment, negotiation with the union may have to occur. If you are not in a unionized environment, you still may have to negotiate with certain individuals to assess gains and losses on both sides. If you have staff members who are absolutely resistant to change, negotiation with these people may include moving the entire group forward and at a faster speed.

You can also co-opt the resisters into the project. Co-option is enlisting the opposing party to help you by giving them a significant role in the process and thereby ensuring their commitment to change. This involves identifying the informal leaders of the group and giving them a significant role in making it happen. But be careful: This strategy can easily be perceived as manipulation, and thereby destroy trust and ensure resistance to anything in the future.

The final approach is coercion. Coercion should be used only as a last resort and when the speed of the project is essential to organizational survival. Coercion is imparting adverse consequences upon staff members who refuse to work toward the change. Although you will see this method described in other areas, it is something to be strenuously avoided because you can risk active movement toward subversion of the plan, which would result in total failure.

Most projects involving change have a date for when the change will be implemented. Once you have established a date for implementation, it is important that you stick to it as closely as possible. People anticipate the change and a certain amount of energy develops in the organization as we move toward the implementation.

If you played a major role in the change or if you are the leader of your unit, it is important that you project a positive attitude regarding the change and see it as opportunity and movement toward progress in the organization. You must be the cheerleader, salesperson, and believer that what will happen is significant for the organization.

LEADERSHIP

TIP

When trying to implement any change, the three most important things to remember are communication, communication, and communication.

You need to continue to keep people informed about progress, and praise those who have helped make it happen. The hardest thing for staff involved in a change is to give up the old ways, unless those old ways were really terrible. During this transition, leaders need to work closely with staff to ensure that they develop the skills they need to make the change successful. If they do not, staff members may get discouraged.

Creating an environment that supports innovation and enhances change

Effective leaders work very hard to help release creative energy within an organization, and staff must understand what is valued in order to support this. When attempting to create an environment that enhances change and supports innovation, you should ask the following questions:

- Does the staff understand what is valued?

- Is there consistency in beliefs and assumptions among those who leave the organization?

- Do people believe that rewards are distributed equally?

- Do management tempers frequently flare up?

- Are management behaviors consistent, or do staff members always have to be alert for the decision of the moment?

- Do you support innovation and change?

- Is your approach consistent, or does it reflect the issue of the moment?

When trying to effect a change, it is occasionally important to seek information and evidence about best practice from outside the organization. Have you sought external advice in the past? If you are able to look objectively at yourself as a leader and at what you value, then you will be more successful as a change agent. Creating a climate of innovation and supporting change when it needs to occur requires a climate in which your staff members are trusted, respected, nurtured, considered, and willing to be challenged. The most important resource you have as a manager is your people. Leaders know that without the people, there is nothing.

To be an effective leader, you need to support innovation and change. Additionally, you need to build information networks that you can use for fact-based problem solving and, above all, you need to understand the rules of your organization and have courage to move change forward. Valuing the diversity and opinions of your people will assist in creating an environment that encourages innovation and change.

Maintaining successful change

Now that the change has been implemented, the environment needs to be monitored and evaluated to see whether the change is achieving the goals that were originally proposed in the plan. Managers must ask the hard questions, which include "Is the change occurring within the allocated time and resources?" and "Are the staff members implementing the new behaviors and processes, or are they backsliding into their old habits and ways of doing things?"

If you thought the work was over once you implemented the change, then you are seriously mistaken. Evaluating and monitoring the change process is probably more difficult than implementing the change itself. When we implement the change, many factors are involved and it is not always possible to anticipate all of the problems that may occur. Additionally, today's healthcare environment, with its rapid changes and decreased resources, leaves little time for proper planning and implementation.

But the basic idea is to plan carefully and be flexible in addressing and adjusting to problems as they arise. Once again, communication is the most important component of our monitoring plan, along with rewarding and reinforcing positive behaviors toward success. For change to be sustained, we need to celebrate the small milestones we achieve, and we need to celebrate the staff members when they bring in ideas that can be implemented. If the change involves a new policy or procedure, it must be constantly reviewed. As we proceed through this process, successes and failures should be documented for future reference and for other teams that might want to implement change.

How can we teach our staff to be effective participants in a change process? As managers and leaders, we know that there is no sure thing and that change is a constant part of our life and of our professional environments. Educating staff in their attitudes and abilities to cope with change can make a difference between success and failure and between satisfaction and dissatisfaction.

Teaching staff to participate in the change process

Here are some tips on teaching your staff how to be successful participants in the change process:

✔ Ask the important questions: who, what, where, when, and why. Understand what the change is and why it should occur. Who is going to benefit and what is required for success?

✔ Look for the benefits of the change, not the negatives.

✔ Offer suggestions and express concerns about the outcomes.

✔ Actively participate, but be patient with setbacks. Participation is the essential ingredient for feeling successful. In the long run, it's not easier to just go along for the ride.

✔ Ask for help, seek support, and remain flexible.

✔ Listen first, speak later.

✔ Celebrate even the smallest success.

Effective project management

As a manager in a healthcare organization, you may find yourself working on projects and will occasionally be asked to lead a project. Sometimes we may be asked to join a project team as part of our regular workday, and sometimes we may be put to work exclusively on a project within the organization.

 A Practical Guide to Leadership Development

> ## Projects
>
> So, what is a project? We could use the word project to describe something that is not necessarily part of your ordinary day-to-day work. It may also indicate something that is purposeful and distinct in character.
>
> Projects contribute to the management of change. A project:
>
> - Has a clear and focused purpose that is achieved within a time frame
>
> - Has a defined beginning and end
>
> - Is established to achieve a specific outcome
>
> - Is usually a one-time activity that is not repeated

You may think that there is no point in carrying out a project if it does not result in change, but change management is the term that usually refers to substantial organizational change, which may include many different types of change in many different areas of work. We discussed some of this earlier in this chapter. Project management, however, refers to one specific aspect of the change. Therefore, projects often have distinct elements that contribute to wider organizational change.

Today's nurse managers find themselves in a role where they administer many small projects at once, every day. Projects in your work environment consist of many different types, including short-term ones such as moving offices, implementing a new form, or organizing a one-time event. Other projects may be bigger, longer, and involve many more people, such as developing a new service or a new function, moving a service area to a new location, or opening a new building. The project you are involved with may deliver an improvement to service or deliver financial benefits to an organization.

Once the project has been defined, it is then possible to estimate what personnel and monetary resources will be needed to achieve the project within the time frame desired. If a pilot project is set up to try out an idea, the outcome for the pilot should achieve its requirements without the need to conduct another pilot project.

Managing a project is different from taking such a role in everyday work simply because of the limited nature of the project. There is a time limit restricting the length of the time that anybody on the project team will be in the role. There are also limits to the type of work produced, and team members are usually selected to bring their expertise to the project for specific reasons. For example, a nurse manager with experience in technology may be asked to assist in the implementation of a new technology project.

When attempting to define a new project, it is very important to set clear objectives that describe exactly what you want to achieve and provide direction for accomplishing that. It is simple to agree to broad goals, but these goals should be translated into specific work objectives if they are going to be used to plan the project.

Objectives should define what is going to be achieved, set a time frame for completion, and determine how the organization will know that the objectives have been met. When writing objectives, the following SMART guidelines should be followed:

- **S**pecific, clearly defined, with criteria for completion

- **M**easurable, so you will know when the objective has been met

- **A**chievable within the current environment, time frame, and budget, and with skill sets that are available from personnel

- **R**ealistic, not trying to achieve the impossible

- **T**ime frame, limited to a completion date and measurement of milestones over the long term

Using measurable objectives in planning your project ensures that you have described what has to be done to achieve the project. However, you should remember that all objectives need to be revisited and revised occasionally, since no plan ever survives the project intact from the beginning. Objectives set early on in the project cycle provide a framework for final evaluation. They also provide information that will help you monitor progress so that the project can be controlled and managed.

 A Practical Guide to Leadership Development

Project parameters and the role of a project manager

There are three key dimensions to any project: budget, time, and quality. All three of these need to be balanced to manage a project successfully. We can call a project successful if it was completed on time and within budget, and if it has achieved the requirements of the project plan. The job of the project manager is to balance all of the dimensions so the project can be managed effectively.

Budget, time, and quality are all linked together, and action on any one of them will affect the other two. For example, if there is a reduction made in the budget, there may be an effect on the amount of time the project takes to complete. If there are fewer people to do the work, then, once again, the time frame and the budget may be affected.

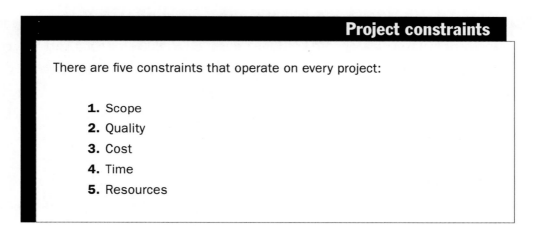

Project constraints

There are five constraints that operate on every project:

1. Scope
2. Quality
3. Cost
4. Time
5. Resources

Scope: The scope of a project is a statement defining its boundaries. It tells when and what will be done. This document is the foundation for the project work that follows because beginning a project on the right foot is important. Also important is staying the course and following the scope of direction. Everyone knows that the scope of a project can change dramatically as the project moves forward. Detecting and reacting to these changes are major challenges for a project manager.

Quality: The quality of a project refers to the quality of the outcome, as well as the quality of the process. It is just as important to focus on how well the project management process works and how it can be improved as it is to look at the outcome. We need to use the process of continuous quality improvement to measure the quality as we move along. Monitoring the quality process and ensuring the process is effective because it increases the probability of successfully completing a project and satisfying all the stakeholders.

Cost: The cost of a project is another variable that defines the project itself. We think of the budget as a set of deliverables that we can provide to the project team. Cost is a major consideration throughout the project management life cycle, and particularly early in the project planning when the budget is developed. However, as contingencies and other issues come up, the budget may have to go up or even down. One of the most important jobs of a project manager is managing the budget effectively.

Time: Time is always our enemy, no matter how well we plan the time frame or deadline in which a project may be completed. There is always some fluctuation. Time is a resource that's consumed, regardless of whether we use it effectively. One of the major objectives of the project manager is to use the time allotted to the project as effectively and productively as possible.

Resources: Resources are connected to time. Once a project has begun, the prime resource available to the project manager to keep the project on schedule, or get it back on schedule, is time. A good project manager realizes this and protects future time very carefully. Other resources include people, equipment, and physical facilities. No matter what resources you have available for your project, they are central to project activities and the project cannot be accomplished without them.

Why projects fail

Projects often fall short of achieving the desired results. This is not due to a lack of efficient project management, but rather from a lack of leadership for that project. Project success is a direct reflection of the person managing it, and it is his or her responsibility not just to manage details and report the status of the project, but to go beyond and add value through project leadership. As someone managing a project, you cannot just update lists, issue meeting minutes, and hold meetings to be successful. Today's complicated healthcare environment requires leaders to take care of projects.

Once again, communication is key to the success of a project. Many groups have interest in knowing project status—for example, the executive management, the implementation team, and the stakeholders—and communication needs to be maintained. Communication with executive management may involve sharing minutes of meetings or just giving informal updates. Communication within a project team is generally informal, consisting of telephone calls, e-mails, and other informal processes to keep the project moving. It is the stakeholders who

A Practical Guide to Leadership Development

usually do not receive the communication as often as they need it. As a project leader, it is critical not to overlook the value of providing regular formal and informal communication with stakeholders.

You may have heard the statement that good planning prevents poor outcomes, and of course it is good planning that facilitates success. However, in business it is the execution of the plan that is the biggest key to success. Sometimes leaders and managers have a tendency to put so much detail into a plan that any deviation from it creates a tremendous amount of work and effort to put the project back on course. We may write the best plan ever, but if we cannot execute it, then we are not going to be successful.

Support from above

Good planning followed by a flawless execution is critical to attaining maximum success in the outcome of the project. In every project you are going to carry out, from the simplest move of an office to the more complicated, such as moving your entire unit into a new facility, you must have the support of top management for it to be successful. But what level of support do we really expect? Sometimes we think the top management is going to be working with us through-out the entire course of the program, and if you, as a project leader, believe that upper management support is critical for your project, then you should aggressively pursue it. Look throughout your organization and find someone in a top management suite who is able to assist you.

Do not blame

As you move along with your project, there may be times when things go wrong, but it is important not to place blame. In project management, it is important to practice the old adage: praise publicly and punish privately. As a project manager, it is your job to make sure that all the changes are successful. When participants in your project have been successful, put them in the spotlight and allow them to share the success and get the credit. It will help build acceptance and ownership of those changes. However, when things go wrong—and they will—you need to focus on solving the problems instead of pointing fingers or accusing other people of failure.

There is no way to plan for every contingency, and things will inevitably not go exactly as planned. As a leader, you will be looked to for advice and help with problems, not to point them out or place the blame. You should accept responsibility to resolve the issues and solve the problems. Solutions begin with you.

As mentioned earlier, the execution of the plan is more important that the plan itself. After you have developed a plan and the focus shifts to the implementation, be careful not to focus too much on the end product and forget about the running of the project itself. All too often, top management is preoccupied with getting to the end and meeting the bottom line. Successful execution of the project is more important, because it will lead to a successful outcome. As a project leader, if you focus on the proper execution of the implementation plan, the results will take care of themselves.

Too often the word "management" implies someone who assigns the tasks, coordinates meetings, and then documents the results. In project leadership, you may need to get right down into the "nitty-gritty" because good project leaders add value to the project by doing work themselves and not simply telling others what to do. There is a balance, however, between doing too much and too little work. Managers must be able to see the big picture. If you are too deeply involved in the project, you lose sight of the scope, direction, and size, and in the end will be ineffective as a leader in trying to move the project forward.

You should behave as if you are in business for yourself, and that it is your money in the project's budget. If it were, you would do whatever it took to make the project succeed, and would not be constrained by organizational functions, boundaries, time constraints, or money to get the job done right.

Every day, you as a frontline manager and leader in your organization are challenged to manage a series of projects in your everyday operation. In many ways, frontline managers today feel frustrated in their inability to complete all of the projects and other issues that they are confronted with on a daily, if not hourly, basis. As a project leader who is trying to manage a series of small projects, it makes sense to share responsibility and ownership with some of those people who are involved in the process on an everyday basis.

Project management alone does not work. Project managers must evolve into project leaders, and by applying some of the strategies discussed in this chapter, you will become a better change agent and project leader. In fact, every change requires some form of project management and leadership. If you as a nurse manager can successfully balance the need for change with the need for effective, efficient, and planned project management, any change you attempt to make in your area or organization will have a much greater chance of success.

 A Practical Guide to Leadership Development

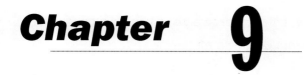

Chapter 9

RETENTION STRATEGIES:
RETAINING THE BEST, LEAVING THE REST

Learning objectives

After reading this section, the participant should be able to:

- Determine factors that contribute to retention
- Discuss the leader's role in promoting retention

Leader's role in retention

In today's rapidly changing and fast-paced healthcare environment, it is important that we look at retention strategies so that we keep our best employees. But it is also important that we work with those who are not the best to improve their performance.

Transformational leadership

There are many simple things you can do as a leader to retain the best staff and make progress toward quality outcomes. One of the newest ideas in leadership is called "transformational leadership." Bass (1985) has described transformational leaders in terms of charisma, inspirational leadership, individualized consideration, and intellectual stimulation. Bennis and Nanus

(1985) indicate that leaders do the right things, whereas managers do things right. In situations like this, leaders focus on effectiveness and managers deal with efficiency.

Leadership strategies

Bennis and Nanus have identified four strategies for taking charge:

1. Attention through vision
2. Meaning through communication
3. Trust through positioning
4. Deployment of self

The leader's vision needs to be clear, attractive, and attainable. Communication through stories, allegories, fables, parables, and analogies helps give meaning to a leader's vision. A leader's visions and positions must be clear because staff are more likely to be trusting when they know a leader's point of view within the organization. Open communication's honesty and consistency are important to building trust. Leaders are continuous learners and use the organization as a learning environment as they deploy themselves and foster a learning environment for their staff.

The idea of transformational leadership has continued to gain in popularity since the early 1980s. Transformational leadership is a process that changes and transforms individuals with emotions, values, ethics, standards, and long-term goals, and concerns itself with assessing followers' motives, satisfying their needs, and treating them as full human beings. Transformational leadership involves exceptional forms of influence, moving followers to accomplish more than they are usually expected to do.

The process of transformational leadership often incorporates charismatic and visionary styles. An advantage to this approach is that it can be used to describe a wide range of leadership, from specific attempts to motivate individuals to broad attempts to influence entire organizations or even cultures. In healthcare, where we are dealing with human beings in most of our interactions, transformational leadership can be extremely effective in retaining your best staff. Transformational leadership is concerned with the performance of followers and also with developing these followers to their fullest potential. Individuals exhibiting transformational leadership often have a very strong sense of internal values and ideals and are effective at motivating followers to act in ways that support the greater good rather than their own self-interest.

In healthcare today, models of transformational leadership are developing throughout our profession. The process of transformational leadership is one in which an individual engages with others and creates a connection that raises the level of motivation and morality in both the leader and the follower. These types of leaders are attentive to the needs and motives of the follower and try to help followers reach their fullest potential.

While we try to retain our best-performing employees, a transformational leadership style may be the one that works best. Because transformational leaders try to help transform individuals from one level to another to help them produce significant and positive change, it is a leadership style that works very well in appealing to a higher level of motivation for individuals. Rather than focusing on tasks, transformational leaders instill in their employees a sense of purpose. Transformational leaders seek to satisfy higher-order needs to fully engage followers by raising the level of consciousness of his or her followers and getting them to reach beyond their emotions to ideals. Followers are thus transformed into better-performing employees, which brings value to themselves as well as to the organization.

While transformational leadership is very powerful and yields significant results, leadership is situational. Effective leaders modify their styles and approach depending upon the situation and what is called for. A research study by McDaniel and Wolf (1992) examined the effects of transformational leadership on work satisfaction and retention of staff nurses. One of the outcomes of the study showed that when transformational leadership was in place, there was positive work satisfaction and low turnover among registered nurses. Despite the limitations of the study (it was a small sample from one institution), transformational leadership produced a positive work environment. In the retention of positive employees, transformational leadership is one style that should be seriously considered for adoption by frontline nurse managers.

Education and retention

Another area that leaders can focus on is staff education. In a 2001 national study released by the Federation of Nurses and Health Professionals, a majority of nurses reported leaving their place of employment because of a lack of education and development. So how do you engage and retain your nurses in an environment where education is expensive, staff is short, it is difficult to allow them to attend education sessions, and they may not be seeking out continuing education? It is important for us as nurse managers to realize that we can either love our staff or lose them. If we love our staff, we treat them fairly and with respect, and we thank them, challenge them, and develop them. If we show that we care about them, we engage and retain them.

On the other hand, the loss is very serious when talent leaves the job, retires, or otherwise disengages from the organization. It is important as nurse managers that we encourage talented people to stay within the organization and especially on our team. Talented and competent nurses are a commodity that must be maintained within an organization.

Focusing on employee development, learning, and growth is a major strategy to keep your most talented nurses. By finding ways to develop workers' talents and enriching their work environment, you allow staff to increase the time that they spend on desirable and innovative work. It is your responsibility as a frontline manager to identify opportunities for employees to move within the organization both vertically and laterally.

Look at the skills of your employees and link them to mentors, coaches, leaders, or colleagues who can offer support and direction for their career development. This can be tough for nurse managers—when we look at an environment that has a shortage of staff, we find ourselves torn between whether or not we really want to assist some of our best and brightest people to move up and out of our unit. But if we do not develop them as individuals, not only will they leave our unit, they will leave the organization as well.

Create a culture that inspires loyalty

Another strategy is to cultivate a style within your unit that inspires loyalty. Ask the staff what they want from their work and what it takes to keep them if they are not happy. Provide feedback; keep them informed; communicate clearly, truthfully, and respectfully; and, above all, listen carefully. Sometimes staff members are not very clear in their perspectives and communication styles. It is your responsibility to understand what they are saying and provide feedback about what you think they are trying to tell you. This can be done by providing a clear direction, identifying and correcting negative behaviors, and looking for meaningful ways to reward them for positive performance.

 A Practical Guide to Leadership Development

Create a work environment with a culture that includes and welcomes diversity, not only differences of race and gender, but thoughts, experiences, and attitudes; this will assist in keeping your staff. Let people take risks and share information freely and regularly. Seek out input from your people. Give them space and provide them the freedom to get the job done in ways that work best for them.

Look for educational opportunities for staff to keep them competent and happy. Since research has confirmed that learning and continuous improvement motivate people to stay with an employer, employee retention specialists concentrate on training and coaching to improve retention at all levels of an organization.

It should be clear in any organization that the retention of staff is everybody's business and not just an issue for the manager, human resources, or training department to fix. By providing a climate where there is a systematic and integrated effort to build employee skills through education and talent, retention becomes a visible and strategic objective.

Organizations need to develop environments in which nurses want to work. By developing that environment, you will have a better chance of retaining your staff. Nurses want to work in safe places that promote quality healthcare. In 2005, more than 40 nurse organizations got together to develop nine principles to help foster staff retention. The Nursing Organizations Alliance™ is a coalition of nursing organizations united to create a strong voice for nurses.

LEADERSHIP

TIP

Visit the Nursing Organizations Alliance Web page at *www.nursing-alliance.org.*

The Alliance provides a forum for identification, education, and collaboration building on issues of common interest to advance the nursing profession. The principles are as follows:

1. Respectful collegial communication and behavior; team orientation; presence of trust; respect for diversity

2. A communication-rich culture that is clear and respectful, open and trusting

3. A culture of accountability in which role expectations are clearly defined and everyone is accountable

4. The presence of adequate numbers of qualified nurses; ability to provide quality care to meet client/patient needs; work and home life balance

5. The presence of expert, competent, credible, visible leadership that serves as an advocate for nursing practice; supports shared decision-making; allocates resources to support nursing

6. Shared decision-making at all levels, in which nurses participate in system, organization, and process decisions; formal structures exist to support shared decision-making; nurses have control over their practice

7. The encouragement of professional practice and continued growth/development, where continuing education/certification is supported/encouraged; participation in professional association is encouraged; an information-rich environment is supported

8. Recognition of the value of nursing's contribution, such as reward and pay for performance; career mobility and expansion

9. Recognition of nurses for their meaningful contribution to the practice

(The Nursing Organizations Alliance, 2005)

Nursing leaders are often put into a role called the "chief retention officer." This position becomes an invaluable liaison between patients, physicians, and other nurses and clinicians. More than anyone else in the hospital, nursing leaders are in a position to create and nurture a workplace culture emphasizing teamwork, communication, and professionalism that ultimately contributes to a sense of job satisfaction. Research suggests that nursing workforce retention increases when nurses are provided opportunities to advance professionally, gain autonomy, and participate in decision-making. There is some evidence to suggest that management styles, such as transformational leadership, flexible employment opportunities, and access to continuing education and professional development, can improve retention of nursing staff as well as patient care.

Leaders need to be mentors and coaches

As a nursing leader, you now have a responsibility to not only be a manager, but also a mentor and coach. One part of coaching and mentoring responsibilities is the education of staff. And, as discussed earlier, we know the education of the staff is a significant item in retaining highly competent people. Coaching and mentoring recognizes that learning occurs most effectively in the process of action. Action learning reflects that the learner is an adult and will experience all that he or she needs to undertake the appropriate role of learner. Coaches and mentors understand that the work environment creates all the opportunity necessary for learning to unfold.

It is important for nurse managers to commit to staff by addressing their learning needs and committing to programs of learning. Leaders can collaborate with educational departments, schools of nursing or universities, or peers within the organization. Nurse managers must recognize the uniqueness of every individual learner and work with appropriate people to develop and implement an individualized learning program for each staff member.

The role of the nurse leader in educating the staff provides an environment for improved patient care. Most staff nurses will engage in self-directed learning to ensure their continued competence. In a self-directed learning environment, it is important that each person knows his or her role: the mentor/coach, the facilitator, or the learner. The basic requirements of the learning relationship include:

- The learner is always in control
- The coach is present for the learner's needs
- The learner is responsible for the outcomes of learning
- The processes of learning are always negotiated
- Coaching is a learning partnership
- The coach is never a "parent"
- Outcomes of learning are defined in advance
- An agreement of learning expectations is always explicit
- The learner determines when the coaching contract is ended
- The coach creates a safe milieu for honest dialogue
- Learning evaluation is performance-based
- Change is always the work of the learner

(Malloch & Porter-O'Grady, 2005)

Coaching involves two-way communication and shows your staff your true ability to learn something about them and their environment in order to improve it. Coaches need to be good listeners who are educated and able to handle conflict resolution. As a coach/mentor you must be familiar with the institution's policies, procedures, and politics. You need to be readily available for the staff and confident in your ability to help them.

Being successful in a leadership position requires you to successfully encourage and support the personal and professional growth of the nurses. Coaching can lead to improved performance and drive excellence through a focus on individual needs. Coaching is about building relationships, setting expectations, and reflecting on their outcomes. Coaches serve to clarify issues and transform problems into action steps and elements of the learning process. A coaching relationship should move toward developing the strengths of each person in that relationship, and while a coach's focus needs to be on the person being coached, the staff member must posses a strong willingness to be coached.

Coaches need to be present and know that the demands on nursing leadership can be frenzied and scattered. When developing relationships with your staff, you have to be willing and able to devote time and energy to develop and maintain relationships. This is a key guideline for developing as a nurse leader, as it is your responsibility to create the environment that will allow your staff to flourish and feel valued. Many a wise mentor has counseled that people don't quit their jobs, they quit their bosses. The boss is the most important person in creating an environment where staff can feel confident, autonomous, and comfortable in what they do. By using the principles of transformational leadership, focusing on nursing education and competence, allowing nurses to practice autonomously, and providing an effective coaching atmosphere, you will create an environment of respect and retain valuable staff. Work with your best; they will help create a positive environment for practice. Those that want to be with you will be very appreciative.

References

Bass, B. M. (1985). *Leadership and Performance Beyond Expectations*. New York: Free Press.

Bennis, W. G., and Nanus, B. (1985). *Leaders: The Strategies for Taking Charge*. New York: Harper and Row.

Federation of Nurses and Health Professionals. (2001). "The nurse shortage: Perspectives from current direct care nurses and former direct care nurses." Opinion research study conducted by Peter D. Hart Research Associates. Accessed at *www.gao.gov/new.items/d01750t.pdf.*

Malloch, K., and Porter-O'Grady, T. (2005). *The Quantum Leader: Applications for the New World of Work*. Boston: Jones and Bartlett.

McDaniel, C., and Wolf, G. A. (1992). "Transformational leadership in nursing service: A test of theory." *Journal of Nursing Administration* 22(2):60–65.

Chapter 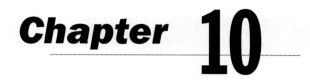 10

SUCCESSION PLANNING

By Alan H. Cooper, PhD, MBA

Learning objectives

After reading this section, the participant should be able to:

- Discuss the benefits of establishing a leadership succession program
- Identify strategies to create the next generation of leaders

Business case for succession planning programs

The role of the leader is to influence others to achieve the goals and vision of the organization. By doing the right things to inspire and motivate the employees to reach these goals and vision, leaders ensure the success of the organization. The most successful companies are those that put the right people with the right skills in the right place at the right time (Ready and Conger 2007).

Since effective leaders are so crucial to success, the importance of developing them at every level of the organization becomes clear. The looming retirement of the baby boomer generation adds further incentive for facilities to ensure that the next generation of leaders is being trained and developed so they will be ready to take the place of today's leaders.

> ## Competent leaders
>
> When developing any leadership development program, care should be taken that leaders are not promoted into positions they are not capable of holding. The Peter Principle, developed by Dr. Laurence Peter, states that members of a hierarchical organization are eventually promoted to their highest level of competence, after which further promotion raises them to a level at which they become incompetent (Peter and Hull 1969). A formal leadership development program should aim to prevent the Peter Principle from being realized by creating competent leaders for the next level.

An argument for establishing a formal leadership development program comes from Jim Collins's classic book *Good to Great: Why Some Companies Make the Leap ... And Others Do Not* (2001). In his book, Collins argues that the jump from a good company to a great company is difficult because "good" organizations are satisfied at that level and it takes extraordinary leadership to become "great." An analysis of the "great" companies Collins discusses in his book shows that only 4.76% of the CEOs of these "great" companies came from outside the organization (Bower 2007). This means that more than 95% of the leaders of these "great" companies are products of an internal leadership development program.

Responsibility for development of the program

Responsibility for succession management and leadership development lies at all levels of the organization. Like other hospitalwide initiatives, leadership development must be driven from the top. Without the support of the senior leadership, including the CEO, leadership development (and all large-scale initiatives, for that matter) is doomed to failure. Responsibility also lies with middle management, department heads, team leaders, human resources, and the staff development function (department, corporate university, etc.). It is extremely important to closely monitor the joint accountability of the program to ensure there are no breakdowns across functions.

LEADERSHIP

Leadership development begins with you and your people. Start identifying your best and brightest today and begin their education.

Hospitals that have the luxury of a corporate university or department of organization development have the advantage of a coordinating body for leadership development activities. Other hospitals may choose to house the coordination function within the human resources department or administration. Regardless of where the program is coordinated, the overall responsibility for the development of future organizational leaders does not fall on one person or one department. It is a shared responsibility throughout the organization that must be taken seriously if the hospital intends on achieving its goals and vision.

Leadership is ongoing

Leadership development is not an episodic or one-time event. You may notice that it is often referred to as a program or process. It is not a "training class" or single occurrence, but rather an ongoing process with cycles of refinement that has multiple aspects and contributors. There are many variations on the theme of leadership development, but most programs build from a unified model. It happens all day every day.

Far too often managers and administrators feel they do not have the time or energy to put into the development of future leaders. The pressures and pace of the daily operation, staffing issues, and financial issues are usually the reasons given for not participating in leadership development. Reasons and excuses range from "I develop my own leaders," to "they learn what they need to know on the job," to "we are too busy to let any of my people go to training classes." These types of excuses are evidence of poor leadership and show a lack of understanding of the leadership development process and leadership in general. Hospital leaders who hear these excuses first need to conduct leadership education for their current staff before they can implement a formal leadership development program.

Choosing candidates for leadership development

The first question to consider is how employees are chosen for involvement in the leadership development program. Are all employees eligible, only current managers, or only those who have been selected as having high potential? The answer to this question will vary based on the needs and resources of the individual hospital or health system. Some organizations, such as GE, focus their leadership development resources on the top 10% of their employees.

Others, such as the North Shore–Long Island Jewish (LIJ) Health System in New York, have created a list of emerging, team, and high-potential leaders drawn from the population of more than 30,000 employees, ranging from frontline staff to current vice presidents, based on criteria created by the senior leadership team.

LEADERSHIP

Think about who could do your job: Who would you want to do it? Who would you want to be your boss?

TIP

The needs of the organization should drive the selection process, and the resources needed, including financial resources, should be considered. A small hospital with limited resources may only need to develop a small number of future leaders, while a large tertiary facility with 6,000 employees may need to develop a greater number. Again, this is an individual decision that should be based on need; there is no magic number or ratio.

The organization should examine its infrastructure and determine what key positions or roles currently need to be filled or may need to be filled in the future, and base its selection decisions on that data. The strategic direction and needs of the hospital should drive the leadership development program and the selection process of candidates.

LEADERSHIP

Think about the right person doing the right job at the right time.

TIP

Once the decision is made as to who is eligible for a succession management or leadership development program, decide on the criteria for entry into the program. A common model is to have senior leaders in the organization nominate candidates based on a set of objective criteria. A single hospital may have each department head nominate candidates based on performance reviews, project success, or other achievements, such as reaching set goals, while senior leaders may nominate department heads based on similar criteria. A multi-hospital health system may use a similar method but also have each hospital head, as well as corporate leadership, nominate candidates. Nominations should be based on objective criteria, and a

A Practical Guide to Leadership Development

team of senior leaders should make the final decisions on the individuals entering the program. Once a list of candidates is developed, it should be reviewed periodically. The list should be dynamic, with candidates being added and removed as the leadership team responsible for the program sees necessary.

LEADERSHIP

TIP

Once people get on the of list of potential candidates, they don't have to stay there. People change and so do circumstances.

Support for candidates

Prior to beginning any formal developmental activities for a candidate, it is important to have a member of the senior leadership team sponsor the candidate. The sponsor is accountable for the success of the candidate and may also act as the candidate's mentor. If a member of the team is not willing to sponsor a candidate, that candidate should be removed from the list (and probably should not have been on it in the first place). The importance and role of mentorship will be discussed later in this chapter.

One approach to aligning succession management and leadership development with the needs of the organization is to create what William Byham refers to as an acceleration pool (2002). Acceleration pools abandon the idea of grooming individuals for specific positions and instead prepare candidates for leadership levels or functions. For example, a hospital may have several levels of acceleration pools, one for frontline supervisors, one for middle managers, and one for senior executives. A hospital could also take the functional approach to acceleration pools. A hospital using this approach might have one pool for nursing, another for ancillary services, and a third for support services. Depending on the size of the organization, these two approaches could be combined with multiple pool levels identified for each function. This approach might be taken by a health system with multiple facilities and services. There are several advantages to the acceleration pool approach. Focusing on levels or functions within the organization instead of individual positions adds flexibility to the program. Another advantage is that it saves senior executives time, since they do not have to match individual development plans with individual positions or fill out replacement planning forms.

The succession management and leadership development process is similar, regardless of whether a hospital uses acceleration pools or an individual position-based development program.

Hire for attitude

A final note about the selection process: It has been said many times by many CEOs, most notably by Herb Kelleher of Southwest Airlines, that it is crucial to hire for attitude and train for skill. This is also true for leadership development programs. Having the right attitude—one of self-development, organizational commitment, customer service, and the desire to make a positive difference—is more than half the battle in becoming a great leader. Attitude plus competency equals performance. Choose the right people, and then develop their competence.

Competency-based vs. competence-based models

The majority of current succession management and leadership development programs use a competency-based model. Healthcare has been moving toward a clinical competency-based model for several years, so this concept should be familiar to most readers. Competencies can be defined as the combination of observable and measurable knowledge, skills, and abilities essential to performing a function, whereas competency can be defined as being adequately or well qualified to perform a task or job. Therefore, a competency-based succession management or leadership development program strives to prepare candidates to be adequately or well qualified for a new position by developing those competencies in individuals that have been identified as necessary for the position, level, or function.

Competency-based programs usually begin by developing a laundry list of competencies that those running the program, or an outside team of experts, feel are important for leadership positions, levels, or functions in the organization. For example, Heller et al. (2004) describe the creation of a nursing leadership development program at the University of Maryland. An advisory board of experienced nurse leaders, in conjunction with project staff and faculty members, identified what they felt were the core competencies for nursing leadership. They identified two types: core knowledge areas and individual leadership skills. Examples of the core knowledge areas included economics and financial management of healthcare delivery systems and managed care; knowledge of technology, patient safety, resource management, and business or administrative practices; and organizational theory and change theory. Examples of individual leadership skills identified included interpersonal skills, communication skills, and organizational navigation. From this list, course objectives were created for the program.

To develop job- or level-specific competencies, teams usually start with a generic list of management and leadership competencies. These lists can be found in various sources, including books and online (visit *www.uscg.mil/leadership/lead/comp.htm* for an example of leadership competencies used by the United States Coast Guard). The list is then narrowed down to include those competencies the team feels a successful candidate must possess for the job or level in question. Detail may be added to specific competencies in order to make them more precise for the job, level, or organization. For example, the generic competency of financial management can be made more specific by changing it to the financial management of healthcare delivery. Once the decision is made on what competencies are needed for the positions, levels, or functions, candidates are evaluated to see which competencies they need to develop or strengthen (see the next section).

LEADERSHIP

TIP

Once you figure out what, then you have to know who. If you compare the who with the what, you'll figure out the competencies people need.

McCall and Hollenbeck (2007) argue that a better approach to leadership development employs a competence model, not a competency model. A competence model uses experiential challenges to develop competence as a leader instead of a list of competencies to be developed. McCall and Hollenbeck state that leadership development (and succession management) should focus on results and not competencies. In a competence model, leaders choose strategically important challenges that will provide developmental experiences for candidates and then help the candidates learn from these experiences. Candidates are reviewed and ranked based on the results of developmental assignments and challenges, not the development of specific skills or knowledge. McCall and Hollenbeck point out that "leaders are forged by the fires of experience" and not by lists of competencies.

It is possible to argue that a competency-based model and a competence-based model are not mutually exclusive. A competency-based leadership development or succession management program must include action learning, stretch assignments, and on-the-job challenges as key developmental experiences. These experiences are created based on the need to develop specific competencies for the individual candidate. A competency-based leadership development or succession management model, however, will include additional learning modalities, such as instructor-led courses, online classes, workshops, and so on. The goal of a competency-based model is to develop competence through multiple avenues, including experiential learning opportunities.

Candidate evaluation

Once the candidates for development have been chosen, they must be assessed for their current level of competency. This can be done in several ways. If the organization has a solid performance management system in place, previous performance reviews can be a good place to start. Reviewing several previous performance appraisals can give a clear picture of the developmental needs of the individual. Additionally, previous performance on goal achievement should be reviewed to identify other developmental needs. Frank conversations with candidates should also take place to discuss what they feel are their needs.

LEADERSHIP

TIP

Good candidates have self-awareness and insight into what competencies they need to develop.

360° evaluations

A 360° evaluation should be used whenever possible to evaluate the candidate's competencies. A developmental 360 begins with the list of competencies the leadership team has developed for the position or level or function. Questionnaires are then distributed, either on paper or online (or sometimes questions are asked in person), asking how the candidate rates on each of the competencies. Usually several questions are asked about each competency, and the results of these questions are rolled up into the overall competency topic. For example, there may be questions on how well candidates speak in public or how clearly they write, which are rolled up into the competency of communication. The questionnaires are filled out by candidates, their direct supervisors, peers, subordinates, and sometimes customers. This way, a clear picture develops on how candidates are perceived on the various competencies by the people around them. If the candidate is an entry-level leader (having no subordinates), the 360 can still be conducted without this group. It would not be considered a full 360, but vital information can still be gained from it.

An important aspect of the 360 results is comparing the scores of the raters. For example, if the candidate's immediate supervisor feels the candidate is weak in an area where the candidate feels he or she is strong, then the blind spot would need further exploration and clarification. The result of the 360 should be a list of the candidate's strengths and weaknesses, and an action plan should focus on areas for improvement. The list of strengths and weaknesses will act as the starting point for the candidate's development plan.

Additional assessment tools may also be used to evaluate candidates entering into the program. The Meyers-Briggs Type Indicator (MBTI) and Emotional Intelligence inventories are two popular assessments used in formal leadership development and succession management programs. The advantage to using these tools is that you get a more robust picture of the candidate. Disadvantages include cost and the need to have the results interpreted.

The 360 results should be combined with the other data discussed earlier, such as operational metrics and other formal assessments, to form an individual development plan for each candidate.

Ideally, a coach should be assigned to each candidate to assist in the interpretation of the 360 results and to facilitate the development of the action plan and the coordination of the developmental learning initiatives. The coach follows the candidate through the process and facilitates his or her development. In the absence of a formal coaching process, a representative from the senior leadership team can assist in these tasks. Coaching education, however, is highly recommended for these individuals prior to working with a development candidate. The coach can monitor and report progress and can thus be useful as a liaison between the candidate and the senior leadership team.

Developmental experiences

The individual development plan must also include the developmental experiences the candidate will take part in to raise the level of the specific competency. Regardless of the type of developmental experience planned, learning objectives must be carefully matched with the competency that the experience is designed to improve. There should be a systematic identification of each learning experience and its alignment with specific competencies.

Developmental experiences

The most common forms of developmental experiences include:

- Internal educational sessions
- External educational seminars or workshops
- E-learning
- Projects or stretch assignments in one's own area of responsibility
- Assignment of articles or books
- Projects or stretch assignments outside of one's own area of responsibility
- Job rotation (moving to a different role or job within the organization)

Since it has been asserted that 20% of corporate learning takes place in the classroom while 80% takes place on the job, a combination of the methods outlined in the list are necessary for success. Stretch assignments and action learning projects have been shown to be the most successful forms of developmental assignments. When candidates lead a team or sponsor a project that is unfamiliar to them, learning must take place in order for them to successfully complete the task. Candidates must also learn where to get vital information to complete assignments.

Different experiences are also important for different levels of employees. For example, a staff employee who is identified as an emerging leader may require internal or external instructor-led classroom time or online education prior to a stretch assignment, whereas a current department head may be sent to a multiday leadership workshop at a college or university or may be given a stretch assignment or become a project sponsor.

Whatever the learning experience assigned, keep in mind that the goals must be aligned with the needs of the candidate and that learning discussions must take place during and after the experience. These learning discussions should link the experience with the specific competency or competencies being developed. The coach or mentor is the ideal person to conduct these discussions.

Coaching and mentoring

The role of the coach and mentor cannot be overemphasized. The coach facilitates the developmental process and keeps candidates on track toward their objectives. An ideal program will have internal or external coaches assigned to each candidate within the program. The coach guides the candidate while providing challenge and support during the development process. Coaches play an integral part in developing and monitoring the action plan, and, as stated earlier, can act as a liaison between the candidate and the leadership team. Coaches also provide the candidate with vital feedback on performance and progress. The use of formally trained coaches within a leadership development and succession management framework is highly recommended.

Mentoring is also a vital part of leadership development and succession management. A mentor, like a coach, acts as a guide for the candidate, but in a role model fashion. A mentor is usually a senior person outside of the formal reporting chain of the candidate and should have regular meetings with the candidate. As previously stated, the candidate's sponsor may also act as his or her mentor.

Importance of mentors

The role of a mentor in leadership development and succession management cannot be overemphasized. However, regardless of the role of the coach or mentor, development is the responsibility of the individual, and the candidate must be held accountable.

Evaluation of progress

Leadership development and succession management is a dynamic process. Candidates need to be evaluated regularly for progress and readiness for their next role. Ongoing evaluation of candidates may be conducted in several ways. For example, follow-up 360 evaluations can be used and compared to the original baseline. This is an excellent way to measure progress since it is a "test, retest" model. The only caveat is that 360s are more subjective than objective and that the raters may change over time.

Other means of evaluation include the objective performance of the leader. Operational measures such as financial performance, employee turnover, efficiency, etc., may be used. Remember, though, that there must be a link between the developmental assignments and the outcome being measured. Some organizations develop an individual scorecard for each candidate to measure progress. Objective metrics are established based on the competencies required. These objectives are regularly measured and then recorded on the scorecard either monthly or quarterly. Like a report card in school, these scorecards can track and trend progress of the individual candidates based on the learning needs identified in the initial evaluation. However, depending on which model of leadership development you are using (i.e., individual or acceleration pools), these scorecards may be different: the metrics may reflect the measures of competencies required for a specific position, level, or function.

Candidates may fall off the development list or progress toward a new position faster or slower based on these evaluations. Development is an ongoing process, and even once competence is reached and a candidate is deemed ready for a specific position, function, or level, development and monitoring does not stop. Continuous assignments and learning opportunities should be provided, regardless of the status of the candidate. Once the candidate is deemed competent for the next position or level, this should be noted by the senior leadership team. When a position needs to be filled, the list should be reviewed for an appropriate candidate. Byham points out that organizations that have researched their succession planning process have found that fewer than 30% of open positions are filled by the person designated as the backup for that position. This fact also points out the advantage of acceleration pools rather than individual position planning.

Leadership development and succession management programs vary in complexity and maturity. Like other large-scale programs, most will start out patchy and will not be broadly accepted. However, if a program is driven from the top, is aligned with the strategy of the organization, and shows consistent successes, it will get buy-in across the board and develop into a successful organizational strategy.

 A Practical Guide to Leadership Development

References

American Association of Colleges of Nurses (2004). "Nursing Shortage Fact Sheet." Available at *www.aacn.nche.edu/Media/Backgrounders/shortagefacts.htm.*

Bower, J. L. (2007). "The CEO within: Why inside-outsiders are the key to succession planning." Cambridge, MA: Harvard Business School Press (as reviewed in *Publishers Weekly*, May 2007).

Buerhaus, P. I., Staiger, D. O., and Auerbach, D. I. (2004). "Trends: New Signs Of A Strengthening U.S. Nurse Labor Market?" Web-exclusive article posted November 17, 2004. *http://content.healthaffairs.org/cgi/content/full/hlthaff.w4.526/DC1.* Accessed 8/4/07.

Byham, W. (2002). "A new look at succession management." *Ivey Business Journal* 66 (5): 10–12.

Collins, J. (2001). *Good to Great: Why Some Companies Make the Leap . . . And Others Do Not.* New York: Harper Business.

Department of Health and Human Services, Health Resources and Services Administration. (2004). "National Sample Survey of Registered Nurses." Available at *http://bhpr.hrsa.gov/healthworkforce/rnsurvey04.*

Health Resources and Services Administration (2007). "The registered nurse population: Findings from the 2004 national sample survey of registered nurses." Available at *http://bhpr.hrsa.gov/healthworkforce/rnsurvey04.*

Heller, B. R., Drenkard, K., Esposito-Herr, M. B., Romano, C., Tom, S., and Valentine, N. (2004). "Educating nurses for leadership roles." *Journal of Continuing Education in Nursing*, 35(5): 203–210.

Lamoureux, K. (2006). "Leadership development maturity model: Executive summary." Bersin and Associates. Available at www.bersin.com/research/leadership_devt.asp.

McCall, M. W. Jr., and Hollenbeck, G. P. (2007). "Getting leadership development right: Help your people to learn from experience." *Leadership Excellence*: 8–9.

McCall, M. W. Jr., and Lombardo, M. M.,(1983). "What makes a top executive?" *Psychology Today:* 26–31

McLure, M. L., Poulin, M. A., Sovie, M. D., and Wandelt, M. A. (2002). "Magnet hospitals: Attraction and retention of professional nurses." In M. L. McClure and A. S. Hinshaw (Eds.), *Magnet Hospitals Revisited.* Washington, DC: American Academy of Nursing.

Peter, L. J., and Hull, R. (1969). *The Peter Principle: Why Things Always Go Wrong.* New York: William Morrow and Company, Inc.

Ready, D., and Conger, J. (2007). "Make your company a talent factory." *Harvard Business Review* 85(6): 68–77.

The Hay Group. (2006). "2006 Best companies for leaders study." McClelland Center for Research and Innovation. Available at *www.haygroup.com.*

 A Practical Guide to Leadership Development

NURSING EDUCATION INSTRUCTIONAL GUIDE

Target audience

- Nurse Managers
- Chief Nursing Officers
- Directors of Nursing
- VPs of Nursing
- Directors of Education
- Staff Development Specialists
- HR Professionals

Statement of need

This book presents an overview of the need for nursing leadership and the challenges of the healthcare environment, and provides guidance for raising the standard of leadership. It discusses leadership competencies and offers practical strategies to help nurse managers on their leadership journey to improve their competence. It also covers how nurse managers and leaders can encourage and develop the next generation of leaders. (This activity is intended for individual use only.)

Educational objectives

Upon completion of this activity, participants should be able to:

- Differentiate between the roles of manager and leader
- Identify three tasks of leadership
- Identify key leadership issues in the healthcare environment
- Identify the necessary competencies for being a healthcare leader
- Describe the benefits of maintaining high standards of professionalism
- Describe the business skill competencies essential for healthcare leaders
- Discuss strategies to improve competence in business skills
- Explain the concept of systems thinking
- Discuss how healthcare leaders can use systems thinking to improve their organizations
- Identify common problems presented by written and verbal communication
- Determine strategies for improving communication
- Examine factors in the healthcare workplace that hinder positive work environments
- Discuss strategies that create a healthy work environment
- Determine how organizational culture and climate affect leadership
- Describe how different leadership styles can be used to suit the situation
- Explain the concept of performance management
- Discuss how leaders can use the concept of performance management to aid the professional development of staff
- Identify ways to resolve performance problems
- Discuss the use of coaching to improve employee performance and development
- Explain how mentors can influence employees' professional development
- Explain the concept of change management
- Examine the role leaders can play as change agents
- Discuss ways to create an environment that supports change
- Explain the role of a project manager
- Determine strategies that will help projects become successful
- Determine factors that contribute to retention
- Discuss the leader's role in promoting retention
- Discuss the benefits of establishing a leadership succession program
- Identify strategies to create the next generation of leaders

A Practical Guide to Leadership Development

Faculty

Dr. Patrick Coonan is the dean and professor of the School of Nursing at Adelphi University in Garden City, NY, and has had a long history of service in nursing service leadership and education. Throughout his career he has held senior patient care management positions at major medical centers in the New York metropolitan area. He has been the chief nursing officer in an academic medical center, a health system, and a teaching community hospital, and completed a fellowship in the Johnson & Johnson–Wharton Fellows Program in Management for Nurse Executives at The Wharton School, University of Pennsylvania. He is certified in Nursing Administration, Advanced, from the American Nurses Association.

Dr. Coonan received his EdD and MEd from Columbia University, a master's in Public Administration/Healthcare Administration (MPA) from Long Island University, and a B.S. in Nursing from Adelphi University. He has written and presented extensively on nursing management, leadership, nursing education, and emergency service and response, as well as healthcare management. His research interests include developing academic/service partnerships, improving patient outcomes, and measuring the impact of leadership, management systems, and nursing care on traditional measures such as complications, costs, and personnel issues.

Alan H. Cooper, PhD, MBA is the vice president for the Center for Learning and Innovation of the North Shore–Long Island Jewish Health System. In this role, Dr. Cooper codeveloped and oversees the leadership development program for a 15-hospital, 35,000-employee integrated health system. He holds an MBA with a concentration in management, and a PhD in experimental psychology with a concentration in human perception and performance. He is an adjunct associate professor at Hofstra University's Frank K. Zarb School of Business and holds a faculty position at the Derner Institute of Advanced Psychological Studies at Adelphi University.

Dr. Cooper is a member of the American Society for Training and Development, the American College of Healthcare Executives, the International Society of Six Sigma Professionals, the American Management Association, the Society for Medical Simulation, and is a senior member of the American Society for Quality.

Accreditation/designation statement

HCPro is accredited as a provider of continuing nursing education by the American Nurses Credentialing Center Commission on Accreditation.

This educational activity for 3 nursing contact hours is provided by HCPro, Inc.

Disclosure statements

HCPro, Inc., has a conflict-of-interest policy that requires course faculty to disclose any real or apparent commercial financial affiliations related to the content of their presentations/materials. It is not assumed that these financial interests or affiliations will have an adverse impact on faculty presentations; they are simply noted here to fully inform the participants.

Patrick Coonan and Alan Cooper have declared that they have no commercial/financial vested interest in this activity.

Instructions

In order to be eligible to receive your nursing contact hours for this activity, you are required to do the following:

1. Read the book *A Practical Guide to Leadership Development: Skills for Nurse Managers*
2. Complete the exam
3. Complete the evaluation
4. Provide your contact information on the exam and evaluation
5. Submit exam and evaluation to HCPro, Inc.

Please provide all of the information requested above and mail or fax your completed exam, program evaluation, and contact information to:

Kerry Betsold
Continuing Education Manager
HCPro, Inc.
200 Hoods Lane
Marblehead, MA 01945
Fax: 781/639-2982

NOTE:

This book and associated exam are intended for individual use only. If you would like to provide this continuing education exam to other members of your nursing staff, please contact our customer service department at 877/727-1728 to place your order. The exam fee schedule is as follows:

Exam quantity	Fee
1	$0
2–25	$15 per person
26–50	$12 per person
51–100	$8 per person
101+	$5 per person

Continuing education exam

Name: _____

Title: _____

Facility name: _____

Address: _____

Address: _____

City: _____ **State:** _____ **ZIP:** _____

Phone number: _____ **Fax number:** _____

E-mail: _____

Nursing license number: _____

(ANCC requires a unique identifier for each learner.)

Date completed: _____

1.   **Which of the following is a key role for leaders?**

   a. Assigning people
   b. Focusing on how to get things done
   c. Focusing on relationships
   d. Working to accomplish tasks

2.   **Which of the following tasks is NOT a task of leadership?**

   a. Communication and relationship management
   b. Developing staff
   c. Being a role model
   d. Budget management

     A Practical Guide to Leadership Development

3. **Which of the following is NOT a key leadership issue?**

   a. Knowing the patient's perspective

   b. Knowing the bed capacity of your facility

   c. Understanding the demographics of the community you serve

   d. Knowing the financial operations of the facility

4. **Which of the following is NOT a necessary competency for healthcare leaders?**

   a. Demonstrating an understanding of the healthcare industry

   b. Knowing the role of nonclinical professionals

   c. Understanding corporate compliance laws

   d. Having a graduate degree in healthcare administration

5. **What is the most important aspect of professionalism that healthcare leaders should possess?**

   a. Ethical responsibility

   b. Financial acumen

   c. Time and stress management techniques

   d. Professional accountability

6. **Why are data collection, analysis, and measurement important to the healthcare leader?**

   a. We collect too much data today and that makes it more difficult to make decisions

   b. Leaders are responsible for the patient's quality outcomes

   c. The data is not important because we have other people who can do analysis for us

   d. Leaders are responsible for keeping all of the paperwork

7. **Which of the following human resource–related strategies will help improve leadership skills?**

   a. Having a working knowledge of policy and procedures, which will help you interpret them for staff

   b. Having in-depth knowledge of all human resource laws and regulations

   c. Attempting to please and accommodate all employees in issues of staffing and scheduling

   d. Entrusting professional development responsibilities to other departments

8. **An example of the feedback loop in healthcare is:**

   a. Root-cause analysis
   b. The personnel management process
   c. Plan, Do, Check, and Act (PDCA)
   d. PCDA

9. **One of the more common problems with healthcare is that unit leaders tend to view:**

   a. Only their unit in regard to management
   b. The entire healthcare organization as integrated
   c. The problems and solutions only on a limited basis
   d. The management and leadership of the organization from a global perspective

10. **Most people only listen to about 50% of what a person is saying to them because:**

    a. They are too busy formulating their response
    b. They don't particularly want to hear what the person has to say
    c. They perceive the information to be incomplete
    d. Most people do not say what they mean

11. **One good strategy to help improve communication is to:**

    a. Look away from people when they are talking to you
    b. Look people in the eye
    c. Shake your head and nod even though you did not hear anything the person was saying
    d. Send more memos

12. **The creation of a positive work environment is important, regardless of whether there is a shortage of healthcare workers, for all these reasons except:**

    a. The work environment affects quality of patient care
    b. The work environment affects the productivity of workers
    c. The work environment affects the financial well-being of the organization
    d. The work environment affects the salary level of employees

A Practical Guide to Leadership Development

13. One strategy that does NOT contribute to a healthy work environment is to:

    a. Put employees first

    b. Develop authentic connections

    c. Coach employees

    d. Encourage gossip

14. Organizational climate has been defined as:

    a. An unconscious pattern of basic assumptions

    b. How it feels to work in a particular environment

    c. Something that can be taught to new members

    d. What the atmosphere is like in any organization

15. The first step in the situational leadership model is:

    a. Coaching

    b. Supporting

    c. Delegating

    d. Directing

16. The concept of performance management concerns:

    a. Efforts to help all employees succeed and improve

    b. Structuring employees' performance

    c. Identifying new financial management systems

    d. Long-term forecasting of patient needs

17. What is the first step in selecting the right person for a job?

    a. Having an appropriate selection process

    b. Having a clearly developed job description

    c. Having clear expectations

    d. Matching skills to job requirements

18. **A good way to ensure that employees are moving in the right direction and to avoid performance problems is to:**

    a. Conduct frequent performance development discussions

    b. Have only two performance improvement meetings per year

    c. Wait until the end of the year and then give the employee his or her performance appraisal

    d. Have informal discussions with the employee in the hallway

19. **One effective coaching technique is known as:**

    a. Recommend, recommend, command

    b. Command, recommend, commend

    c. Commend, recommend, commend

    d. Commend, recommend, command

20. **Mentor relationships can happen in:**

    a. Formal environments

    b. Informal environments

    c. Both formal and informal environments

    d. Neither formal nor informal environments

21. **Changes occur in organizations as a result of forces that affect the organization, both internally and externally, and these forces can act on individuals or the organization as a whole. A leader's role in change management is to be a:**

    a. Change neutralizer

    b. Change blocker

    c. Change agent

    d. Change damper

22. **A key role for leaders as change agents is to:**

    a. Assess the difficulties or problems that the change is designed to alter

    b. Assess the patient care situation

    c. Assess their own leadership style

    d. Assess regulatory implications

23. **When creating an environment that supports change, leaders have to understand employees' feelings toward change. The hardest thing for employees to do is:**

    a. Give up the old ways

    b. Understand all the possibilities of change

    c. Make the transition from old to new

    d. Develop new skills

24. **What are the three key dimensions to any project that project managers must consider?**

    a. Quantity, time, budget

    b. Time, budget, scope

    c. Quality, time, budget

    d. Scope, time, quantity

25. **The primary reason projects fail is because:**

    a. There was not enough money

    b. The scopes were written poorly

    c. The person running it failed to manage it appropriately

    d. The original plan was written poorly

26. **A major strategy to keep your most talented nurses is:**

    a. Giving them raises twice a year

    b. Focusing on development, growth, and education

    c. Identifying opportunities for advancement

    d. Giving them every weekend off

27. **The leader's role in coaching and mentoring recognizes that learning occurs most effectively:**

    a. When there is an environment of learning

    b. When coach and mentor meet regularly

    c. When the work environment is negative

    d. During the process of action

28. **Why is it important that candidates in a succession plan have a sponsor from the senior leadership team?**

    a. Because you can't be in the budget without one

    b. Because they are accountable for the candidate's success and serve as their mentor

    c. Because having a senior leadership sponsor its credibility to the candidate

    d. Because they will be removed from the list unless they have one

29. **Strategies to promote the next generation of leaders include developing job- or level-specific competencies. How can this help succession planning?**

    a. Candidates can be evaluated to see which competencies they need to develop or strengthen

    b. Candidates can apply the competencies to further education

    c. Candidates can evaluate which candidates are more qualified than themselves

    d. Candidates can choose to apply for other positions

A Practical Guide to Leadership Development

Continuing education evaluation

Name: _____

Title: _____

Facility name: _____

Address: _____

Address: _____

City: _____ State: _____ ZIP: _____

Phone number: _____ Fax number: _____

E-mail: _____

Nursing license number: _____

(ANCC requires a unique identifier for each learner.)

Date completed: _____

1.   **This activity met the learning objectives stated:**

     Strongly Agree   Agree   Disagree   Strongly Disagree

2.   **Objectives were related to the overall purpose/goal of the activity:**

     Strongly Agree   Agree   Disagree   Strongly Disagree

3.   **This activity was related to my continuing education needs:**

     Strongly Agree   Agree   Disagree   Strongly Disagree

4.   **The exam for the activity was an accurate test of the knowledge gained:**

     Strongly Agree   Agree   Disagree   Strongly Disagree

5. **The activity avoided commercial bias or influence:**

    Strongly Agree   Agree   Disagree   Strongly Disagree

6. **This activity met my expectations:**

    Strongly Agree   Agree   Disagree   Strongly Disagree

7. **Will this activity enhance your professional practice?**

    ❏ Yes   ❏ No

8. **The format was an appropriate method for delivery of the content for this activity:**

    Strongly Agree   Agree   Disagree   Strongly Disagree

9. **If you have any comments on this activity please note them here:**

    _____

    _____

    _____

    _____

    _____

10. **How much time did it take for you to complete this activity?**

    _____

Thank you for completing this evaluation of our continuing education activity!

Return completed form to:

HCPro, Inc. • Attention: Kerry Betsold • 200 Hoods Lane, Marblehead, MA 01945

Telephone: 877/727-1728 • Fax: 781/639-2982